Keto Diet

+

Intermittent Fasting

+

Mediterranean diet

3 in 1

Essential and Definitive Weight Loss Guidefor Women and Men, New Mini Healthy Habits, Ketogenic Lifestyle and Reverse Disease

By Serena Baker

2

Table of Contents

Additionally, the information in the following pages is intended only for informational purposes and should thus be thought of as universal. As befitting its nature, it is presented without assurance regarding its prolonged validity or interim quality. Trademarks that are mentioned are done without written consent and can in no way be considered an endorsement from the trademark holder.

Keto Diet for Beginners:

Easy and Complete Weight Loss Guide to a High-Fat/Low-Carb Lifestyle.

Reset your Health With these Ketogenic-Fasting Ideas, and add more Clarity and Confidence in your Life!

By Serena Baker

Introduction

Congratulations on beginning your journey to weight loss, health, and feeling great! At first glance, the ketogenic diet seems overwhelming and complicated. People think it's not something they can stick with, or share with friends and family. But the reality is it's a lot easier than you think! In this book, we are going to hold your hand and take you step-by-step through the ketogenic diet. First, we'll give an overview of what the diet is and how it works. Then we'll review the benefits of the diet. After we've got all the basics covered, we'll tell you exactly what you need to know in order to get started! We'll give you an eating plan and recipes. Not sure what to eat for breakfast? We've got you covered! And lunch and dinner too.

The ketogenic diet is quite easy to follow. It seems like a diet you won't be able to fit in with your friends when they want to go out to eat, but nothing could be further from the truth. If you're just a little bit careful, following the keto diet (as it's known for short) is very easy. So, let's get started!

Chapter 1: An Overview of the Ketogenic Diet

If you're like me, then for years you've been completely brainwashed. Nutrition experts, doctors, and dieticians all said the same thing – Eat a low-fat diet! They told us that fat put the weight on, raised our cholesterol, and caused heart attacks.

A funny thing happened – none of that turned out to be true. After years of telling everyone that they needed to eat a high-carbohydrate and low-fat diet, doctors began noticing something strange. People were putting on weight! And nobody was getting any healthier. At first, they thought it was because people couldn't stick to diets. And there was some truth to that. After all, dieting using the old scheme required calorie counting and deprivation. Most of us found that got old fast. When the hunger pains came, we dove in.

Finally, it began dawning on people maybe something wasn't right. Years ago, Dr. Atkins had been urging people to eat low carb. Some were doing it, but the vast majority of doctors thought it was nutty. But as the experts started learning about diabetes and the way the body worked, they began to realize that Atkins was onto something and that the low-fat diet idea was wrong.

What Is the Ketogenic Diet?

The ketogenic diet is a high-fat, moderate-protein, and low-carb diet. There's nothing very complicated about it. It's a little bit different, than the standard low-carb dieting you've heard about, because generally people on low-carb haven't worried about their protein intake. With keto, you eat proteins in adequate amounts but keep them in check. We'll see why that's the case in a bit.

But what about all that fat? Is it going to clog my arteries?

The answer for most people is a resounding *no*. The ketogenic diet is based on a diet of healthy fats. You probably already know the standard litany – omega-3's in fish, and olive oil are right for you, but animal fat, not so much.

Well, guess what. That turned out not to be true either.

Yes, it is true that olive oil is right for you. And so are fish. But what about animal fat? Well about five years ago or so researchers got a big shock. When the saturated fat found in animal meats was studied in detail – they found out it didn't raise heart attack risk at all.

So, it's safe to eat a fatty cut of steak. In fact, we encourage it. Basically, you can think of saturated fat as the neutral fat, and olive oil and fish oil are the best fats. It turned out that saturated fat only causes health problems when it's consumed in a diet heavy on carbs. When you're eating low carb, it's just fine. So, go ahead and have some steak and lamb, and add some butter if you want to.

The History of the Ketogenic Diet

The ketogenic diet traces its roots to the treatment of epilepsy. Surprisingly this goes all the way back to 500 BC, when ancient Greeks observed that fasting or eating a ketogenic diet helped reduce epileptic seizures. In modern times, the ketogenic diet was reintroduced in the practice of medicine to treat children with epilepsy. In 1921, a scientist named Rollin Woodyatt discovered that the liver made ketone bodies during starvation or when the patient was following a high fat, low carbohydrate diet.

Research into the keto diet stalled until the 1960s, when scientists discovered that a certain class of fats called *medium chain triglycerides* or MCTs were readily transported to the liver and made into ketone bodies, faster than normal fats (coconut oil is an example). It was also found that the body could go into a state of ketosis eating more protein when large amounts of MCTs were consumed.

In the early 1970s, a cardiologist named Robert Atkins proposed his own version of a ketogenic diet called the Atkins diet, which has been immensely popular. The Atkins diet has more relaxed standards that keto, allowing adherents to follow very strict carbohydrate consumption for the first two weeks during an "induction phase." After this, the number of carbohydrates consumed can be slightly increased.

From there, research on ketogenic diets stalled again. However, in the past fifteen years, there has been an explosion of interest in the diet.

How Keto Is Different from Other Diets

It's obvious how keto is different from many diets. The standard American way of dieting is to eat a high carb diet while restricting fats. Extensive calorie counting is required. It can be said that the keto diet is the opposite of the standard method of dieting.

Another popular diet is the Mediterranean diet. This diet, which is based on the eating habits of people who live along the Mediterranean Sea, is based on a varied diet including fish, whole grains, nuts, fruits, vegetables, cheese, and occasional meat. Legumes also play a central role in the menu. Many health benefits are ascribed to the keto diet but it still involves the consumption of large amounts of carbohydrates, so may not work well for those who are attracted to the keto diet.

There are many other low carbohydrate diets on the market. We've already mentioned the Atkins diet, which has been very popular and kept the keto-eating pattern alive in the public mind. The keto diet is stricter than Atkins. As we mentioned above, Atkins allows dieters to limit carbohydrate consumption to 20 grams a day for the first two weeks. After that, they can gradually add more carbs to their diet up to a point. The keto diet is different in that you cannot start adding carbs to the diet. Some people may find they do better eating carbs at a higher level, but generally speaking, a keto diet is a lifestyle change rather than a temporary "diet." Another difference between keto and Atkins is that Atkins doesn't place formal limits on protein intake; its focus is only on limiting the number of carbs consumed daily.

The *Paleo diet* claims to be based on the eating patterns of pre-historical peoples. Whether this is true or not we'll leave to the anthropologists to figure out, but paleo (and an offshoot known as "primal") is a style of low carb eating that is someone more relaxed than Atkins and ketogenic dieting. Paleo allows the consumption of specific high fiber but high carb foods like sweet potatoes that are not allowed on keto. Many paleo adherents also eat nuts and berries, which adds more carbs to the diet than what would probably be considered appropriate on keto. However, the paleo diet is quite a change from the standard American diet.

The South Beach Diet is another low carb diet, which is really an offshoot of the Atkins diet. The difference is Atkins, at least as initially proposed, allow people to eat any amount of fat they like. South Beach attempted to combine the popular notion of eating lean proteins with a low carb diet. It works for some people, but if you are trying to get by on low carbs with low-fat meals, you'll probably find yourself hungry, lacking mental clarity, and feeling unsatisfied.

On the other end of the spectrum, we have the *Ornish* diet, vegetarians, and veganism. The Ornish diet takes standard dieting advice to the extreme, favoring low glycemic carbohydrates in large amounts and severely restricting fat intake, to less than 10% of calories.

At first sight, the vegetarian and vegan diets might seem the opposite of keto, but in fact, you can be a vegetarian and still enjoy a keto diet. The hard part is getting vegetarian protein sources that are also low in carbs. However, many oils can be safely consumed like olive oil, and you can eat all the avocados you like.

The Science Behind the Ketogenic Diet

Researchers are starting to build a large amount of evidence that supports the ketogenic diet. In 2004, an article titled "Long-term effects of a ketogenic diet in obese patients" was published in Experimental Clinical Cardiology. The researchers found that a 24-week diet that limited daily carbohydrate intake to 30 grams and total protein intake to one gram per pound of body weight resulted in significant weight loss among participants. The patients in the study also saw improved lipid profiles, with increasing HDL or "good" cholesterol and decreased levels of LDL or "bad" cholesterol, triglycerides, and blood sugar. Later researchers have confirmed that a ketogenic diet leads to significant weight loss when studied in a controlled setting, while also providing other benefits such as better blood sugar control.

What Are the Health Benefits of a Ketogenic Diet?

The first benefit of the ketogenic diet is weight loss. When you start keto, if you actually stick to it, you're going to lose weight rapidly. With no carbs to burn for fuel, your body turns to burn fat – including *your fat*. And for reasons that we'll explain in a minute, you'll also get rid of unwanted water weight.

If it stopped there, the keto diet would be a wondrous thing. But we're just getting started – the keto diet has many benefits. First, let's talk about diabetes.

In many western societies, especially in the United States, diabetes is at epidemic levels. The culprit is our diets – and it's not what they thought it was. You're probably guessing by now it wasn't fat, *it was the carbs*. For people with the genetic tendency, eating a carbohydrate diet made them gain weight and set them up for diabetes.

That's where the keto diet comes in. Health benefit number two is it lowers your blood sugar and often does so dramatically. If you're pre-diabetic or diabetic (type 2), you may be shocked with the results you get doing keto. Your fasting blood sugars are going to drop, and you'll see lower A1c scores as well. For some, they've even dropped into the normal range. If you're pre-diabetic and not on any meds, you can probably manage this yourself. But if you already have diabetes and take medications, be sure to discuss your keto eating plan with your doctor. Your dropping blood sugar might mean you need to dial back your medications or insulin.

Speaking of insulin, many people who don't have diabetes develop insulin resistance as they become middle-aged. They get a little pudgy around the middle, and when they eat a high carb meal, their cells just don't work right. The pancreas releases the insulin it's supposed to, but the cells don't quite respond. They've become *insulin resistant*. More insulin needs to be released to get them to take up the sugar. The good news is a keto diet will lower insulin resistance.

Another benefit of the keto diet is that directly lowers your risk of heart disease. Crazy right? Eating all that fat and you have a *lower* risk of heart attack? That almost seems like a magic trick. Here's how it does it – triglycerides. While doctors were fretting about total cholesterol, they didn't notice all those people with normal cholesterol levels having heart attacks. What was going on?

First a brief overview of blood fats. Cholesterol is transported through the body using *lipoproteins*. This is a molecule made up of fat ("lipo") and protein. There are two significant types of cholesterol you need to be concerned about, which are classified by their density, or how crowded they are packed. One is low density or LDL, and the other is high density, or HDL. Traditionally we've been told that a high cholesterol number is not good for you, but after decades of research, scientists have discovered that this designation is simplistic. Half of all first time heart attack victims have supposedly healthy levels of total cholesterol.

LDL was believed to be the culprit behind heart disease, and this is true to a degree, but the picture is not as simple as once believed. However, the legacy belief that its bad for you has led to the designation that LDL is "bad cholesterol." For years, doctors have believed that just by controlling LDL levels, they could reduce heart disease risk.

It turns out that there are many risk factors for heart disease, and one little-noticed lipid problem is the amount of triglycerides in your blood, which is a type of blood fat. More specifically, your heart disease risk is accurately determined from the ratio of triglycerides to HDL.

Triglycerides are blood fats the liver makes after a meal, usually one heavy in carbohydrates. A large amount of triglycerides are also produced by the liver when an excess amount of alcohol is consumed.

HDL is also known as "good cholesterol." Its job is to clean out excess LDL or "bad cholesterol" from the arteries. Next time you get blood labs done get your numbers and do a little calculation if they don't do it for you. Divide your triglyceride number by the HDL number. If it's less than three, you're OK. Ideally, it should be close to one. However, if it's greater than three, you have a high risk of having a future heart attack.

Luckily the keto diet steps up to the plate again. When you follow a keto lifestyle, you'll see your triglycerides drop. Many people see utterly dramatic results. For many, HDL also increases. So, keto will lower your triglyceride to HDL ratio and dramatically decrease your risk of heart attack.

If that were all keto did, we'd be happy, but it turns out higher insulin levels in the body can also raise blood pressure. That's a terrible thing – high blood pressure can lead to many serious health problems. It raises your risk of stroke and heart attack, as well as putting you at risk for kidney damage and other issues.

One reason this happens is raised insulin levels can cause water and salt retention. And that leads to high blood pressure. The good news is that by lowering your insulin levels, keto leads to lower blood pressure values in many people.

Insulin also acts as a fat storing hormone. When you're eating a high-carbohydrate diet, all that insulin flowing around is going to tell your body to store the sugar in fat cells. This is how high carbohydrate diets can make people gain weight even if they are eating low fat and "watching the calories." If we keep blood sugars stable and level, there is less insulin released, and as a result, the body will store less fat. The healthy way to achieve this result is to eat a keto diet.

Keto has also been shown to improve mental health. This isn't surprising, for nearly a century it's been used to treat epilepsy in children. So, doctors have known for some time that keto diets had an impact on the nervous system. Now many people are reporting more stable moods, less depression, and higher concentration on keto.

Keto diets can also help with sleep and digestion problems. The reason for this is that the blood sugar spikes that you get while on a typical western diet high in carbs won't be happening anymore. With keto, your blood sugar will be steady as she goes at all times. This also helps with mood and anxiety as well.

Ketosis: A Detailed Overview

Usually our bodies use sugar for energy. Blood sugar rises after a meal is digested, and then insulin is released. Insulin tells your cells to take up the sugar. You can think of insulin as a signal or as a key that opens a door. Once the cells take up the sugar, they can process it to obtain energy and your blood sugar drops back down to background levels.

As we age and gain weight, our cells become insulin resistant. This means that they are less responsive to the hormone insulin, so won't take up as much sugar. The blood sugar in the body rises, and this creates a large number of health problems. Blood sugar can damage your blood vessels and left unchecked high blood sugar levels can cause kidney failure, blindness, heart disease, stroke, and other problems like erectile dysfunction.

Early on there probably aren't any symptoms at all, and you'll only notice that you're putting on weight every year. Maybe you feel a little more fatigued, and if it continues to get worse, you might find yourself drinking more water.

As insulin resistance develops, the body tries to compensate by releasing more insulin. This sets up a deadly cycle. Over time more and more insulin needs to be produced to keep up.

To avoid the deadly cycle, we can rely on metabolizing fats instead. It turns out that sugar isn't the only fuel the body can run on. When you're either fasting or your body is low on sugar, the body can produce fuel from another source by burning fats for energy. This process is called *ketosis*.

Ketosis works by using three molecules that scientists call acetoacetate, beta-hydroxybutyrate, and acetone. If that gave you a momentary headache don't worry about it! To understand ketosis you don't have to know the actual names of the molecules. All you need to know is that the body can utilize these three ketones for energy in place of sugar. When ketones are found in the blood, the body is said to be in a state of *ketosis*.

Under certain circumstances, the liver will convert fat into ketones. When the liver releases ketones, they enter the bloodstream and are distributed throughout the body where they can be used by the cells as fuel.

Something important to know is that too much protein will inhibit this process. This is because the body can make glucose (blood sugar) from protein, and it will do so when actual sugar is in short supply. Overeating protein is often a reason that people "hit a wall" when attempting low-carb diets such as Paleo or Atkins. They eat too much protein and end up keeping their blood sugar levels high, and fail to enter ketosis. The result is they are unable to lose weight.

So, keep this rule in mind: eat adequate protein but only eat protein in moderation.

The question before us is how do we put the body into a state of ketosis. The way to do it is to deplete your sugar levels. The uncomfortable way to do it is to go through a period of fasting. When you're not eating anything, you're not eating carbs either, and you'll go into ketosis. Some people do incorporate fasting into their keto program, and that may be an option for you. However it's not necessary, and you can still achieve the same results without starving yourself.

How? By eating a diet with moderate amounts of proteins, very low carbs and high levels of fats – we naturally put the body in a state of ketosis.

While you don't have to do it, many people are interested in actually finding out if they are in ketosis. You can buy and handheld meter and find out. The meter will report the level of ketones in your blood. Ketones are measured in units of mmol/L. It is recommended that your ketone level is in the range of 1.5-3.0 mmol/L. This is the "optimal" range which will help you achieve your weight loss goals. If your ketone level is below this range, then you need to take a closer look at your diet.

First, make sure you're not eating too much protein. If that isn't the culprit, then look at your total carbs and see if you can reduce them.

A ketone test kit can be purchased online for around $50-$70.

People doing keto for the first time may experience some unpleasant side effects when going into ketosis. The most common symptoms are feeling "under the weather." Some people call this the "keto flu," and it's characterized by lethargy, possible headaches, and irritability. Some people will also experience constipation, and others may experience heart palpitations.

The best way to avoid these problems is to do the following: make sure you're getting enough water and enough key minerals. You may need to drink more water than you're used to, at least at first. Other problems, in particular, heart palpitations, maybe caused by a failure to get adequate minerals. Two key minerals you should focus on are potassium and magnesium. You can take supplements, but the problem with potassium is that they only come in 99 mg pills and the daily requirement is in the thousands of mg. The best way to get potassium is from your diet. Meat does supply some potassium, and you can also get it from leafy green vegetables and broccoli. If you find out or feel your potassium level is low, consider adding spinach, arugula, or kale to your eating plans.

You can use magnesium supplementation. It is often available in 250 mg or 500 mg doses. You'll want to take a maximum of 500 mg per day. Magnesium helps a great deal with heart palpitations, maintaining proper blood pressure, and avoiding constipation.

But here's a tip. Eat avocados. This lush fruit is mostly fat, and it's mainly good monounsaturated fats. But for our purposes here the key fact about avocados is that they contain ample amounts of vitamins and minerals. Checking the nutrition facts, we find that one cup of sliced avocado supplies 24% of your vitamin c needs, 20% of vitamin B-6, 10% of magnesium, and 20% of daily recommended potassium. That cup of avocado only has 2 grams of net carbs as well – so it fits in with a keto diet.

That brings up an important aside, how do you calculate net carbs? It's very easy. Only note the total carbs and the dietary fiber. Subtract dietary fiber from total carbohydrates. That's the net carbs for any food.

Now let's turn to a thorny issue – *ketoacidosis*. First, let's be clear that ketoacidosis is not something you have to worry about at all. But we have to bring it up because it sounds like ketosis and people often confuse the two processes. But they are not the same and are not caused by similar processes. Ketosis is a normal process used by the body. Ketoacidosis is a dysfunctional situation.

First off, ketoacidosis is only of concern for diabetics – and chiefly those with type 1 diabetes. If you don't have type 1 diabetes, you shouldn't be worrying about ketoacidosis.

Ketoacidosis is a malfunction that occurs when the level of ketone bodies in your system reaches 10-15 mmol/L. This can cause stomach pain, nausea, and vomiting. Higher levels can result in confusion and even coma or death.

However, when you're following a ketogenic diet, you're likely to max out at a ketone body level of 3 mmol/L, a level much lower than that seen with ketoacidosis. Reasonably healthy people can maintain levels of ketone bodies within safe levels very easily. This is because your pancreas will release insulin if ketone bodies get too high, and this will signal the liver to stop making them.

That's why type 1 diabetics have to worry about ketoacidosis. Their bodies can't produce insulin, so could not shut down a runaway ketone body problem. For most of us, this is not something we need to worry about.

However, there are two cases where ketoacidosis could be a concern even if you don't have type 1 diabetes. This is when you have type 2 diabetes and taking certain medications, or you're breastfeeding. If you're breastfeeding, you may want to discuss a keto diet with your doctor first. Complications with breastfeeding and keto are rare, however.

In the case of type 2 diabetes, those taking the medications Farxiga, Jardiance, or Invokana (or other SGLT-2 inhibitors) may be at risk of ketoacidosis if they go on a ketogenic diet. If you have type 2 diabetes and taking one of these drugs, please speak to your doctor first. It may be important to discontinue the medication before going on a diet.

In any case, if you're breastfeeding or a person with type 2 diabetes taking one of these medications and you suspect that you're showing the symptoms of ketoacidosis, eat some carbohydrates. This will help release insulin and stop the process. Then call 911. It's also good to have a ketosis meter on hand so you can check your blood level of ketones.

A surprising fact about ketones is that they're brain food. Many people (including some doctors) mistakenly believe that the brain must have blood sugar for energy. The truth is that is not the case. The brain is perfectly happy burning ketones for power, and there is some evidence that this is better for the brain. Ketone bodies may help the brain function better and stabilize moods.

To maximize weight loss, you'll want to optimize ketosis. This means that you should have ketone bodies in the range of 1.5-3.0 mmol/L. If you are in the range 0.5-1.5 mmol/L, you're said to be in "light ketosis." That's better than not being in ketosis at all, but you want it in that 1.5-3.0 mmol/L range. If you're not in the optimal range first, make sure your carb intake is as low as you want it to be. It's a good idea to keep a journal or record of your food consumption, so you know exactly how many carbs you're consuming. You'll also want to note the number of grams of protein per day, since overeating protein will result in the liver making glucose, raising your blood sugar levels. This will inhibit ketosis and inhibit weight loss.

Determining If Keto Is Right for You

You wouldn't be reading this book if you weren't interested in losing weight and improving your cardiovascular health. But is keto for everyone? It turns out it's not, but keto should work out for most people. The best way to determine if keto is right for you is to see if you are one of the people who *shouldn't* be on keto. If you're not in one of those groups, then keto is right for you after all. So, who are the people that shouldn't be on keto? There are no hard and fast rules, but we can consider the following:

- High blood pressure. If you have high blood pressure keto may not work for you. However, it will probably work out fine for most people with high blood pressure, in fact, it will probably help them get off their medications by causing weight loss and also some loss of body fluids and the associated excess salt. But you should realize that keto can lower your high blood

- pressure, and if you're on medications that can cause some problems. You should discuss this with your doctor. If you start keto and your blood pressure drops, your doctor may have to adjust your medication dosage. But that's what we're hoping for anyway!

- Breastfeeding. In rare cases, breastfeeding moms can run into trouble while on keto. Discuss with your doctor first.

- People with type 2 diabetes. With type 2 diabetics, there are two areas of concern. Your blood sugar levels may drop eliminating the necessity of medications like metformin. If you're using insulin, dosages will need to be reduced or even eliminated since you're not consuming carbs. As noted above, if you're taking an SGLT-2 inhibitor like Farxiga, you may be at risk of ketoacidosis. In all cases speak with your doctor about these issues before doing a keto diet.

- People with type 1 diabetes.

If you're not in one of those groups, then you should be good to go with a keto diet. The only issue once we've cleared up possible health risks is making sure that you're disciplined enough. Are you unable to give up carbs, period? If so, then maybe the keto diet isn't for you. That doesn't mean you can't have an occasional lapse or even now and then cheat day, but those who want to keep eating everything probably shouldn't go on keto. Do you value potato chips and the occasional slice of bread or losing weight more? Ask yourself and then act appropriately.

Pros and Cons of the Keto Diet

Quite frankly the advantages of the keto diet are easy. We've already discussed many of them. Let's list them here:

- You'll lose weight and look better.
- Lose body fat.
- More energy.
- Mental clarity.
- Stable moods.
- Risk of heart disease will drop.
- Risk of stroke will drop.
- Risk of some cancers related to obesity will drop.
- You'll sleep better.
- You'll reduce acid reflux if you have it.
- You'll reduce acne if you have it.
- Blood sugar will be reduced.
- If you're pre-diabetic, you'll probably cure it.
- If your diabetic you'll probably cut your A1C, and some may be able to get off medication.
- Your blood lipids will improve.
- If you're suffering from non-alcoholic fatty liver disease, going on keto will cure it.
- You'll think less about food.
- A keto diet may reduce the risk of cancer.

That's a long list, and we've probably missed a few things. But we'd be lying if we said that keto was the perfect diet. There are some cons of the keto diet.

- Lethargy or headaches. Most likely due to "keto flu." Make sure you're drinking enough water. Also, check your mineral intake.

- Dry mouth. Results from not enough water. It's sometimes recommended to drink a cup of bullion each day, to help your body maintain proper salt levels (remember keto causes fluid loss, salt goes with it).

- Increased urination. When you first adapt to keto, you might urinate more than usual. This effect is usually temporary.

- Bad breath. This results from acetone in your breath and sometimes in your sweat. Usually temporary.

- Reduced exercise performance. If you're a pro-athlete, you may have issues with reduced performance from a lack of carbs.

So, what's the verdict? We vote yes on the keto diet. Most of the downsides are minor and temporary.

Issues That May Come Up with a High Fat Diet

Most issues that come up with a high fat diet like keto result from beginners' mistakes. Your body is used to balance it gets via minerals and fiber in foods like pasta and bread. When you suddenly stop eating these foods, without adequate replacements you may run into issues.

One of the most common issues that comes up on a high fat diet like keto is constipation. There are three main reasons for this that you can look into if this happens to you. The first is to make sure you're getting adequate water intake. The second issue you may face is not getting enough fiber. To increase fiber, look at adding some low carb vegetables to your meal plans. Spinach, kale, arugula, cauliflower, and broccoli are excellent choices. You may also consider avocado, which is packed with both fiber and essential minerals. But please be aware of the calories contained in avocado. Finally, check your magnesium.

Heart palpitations are a common problem for beginners in high-fat diets. Typically, these result from an easily corrected mineral imbalance. The usual culprit, in this case, is magnesium. You can either address it by adding magnesium-rich fruits and vegetables to your diet or by using supplements.

Irritability and brain fog are also common complaints when starting keto. Usually, these are temporary problems as your body adjusts. If they continue to make sure your water intake and minerals are where they need to be.

Muscle loss is an unexpected issue that may come up with some keto dieters. While it's important to consume protein in moderate quantities, some people end up eating too little protein. Make sure you get adequate amounts of protein, especially if you're someone who works out.

Tips and Tricks for Transitioning to a Keto Lifestyle

Now let's have a look at some tips that will help you adapt to a keto lifestyle successfully. The first thing to remember is that for most people, this style of eating is a significant change in their lives. So, the first thing you need to bring to the table is a firm commitment to losing weight and improving your health. If you're the kind of person who is going to be easily tempted by cheating, the keto lifestyle may not be for you. But if you've committed, let's forge ahead.

One tip is to get a friend to go on keto with you. It helps to have a support system, and while you can (and should) get online to talk to others also starting on a keto diet for support and to exchange ideas, it helps to have a personal friend involved. You may already have some friends trying out a keto diet or others who are thinking about it. Talk to them and find out. If you can do it together the added support will help you stay on a diet.

Next, make sure you familiarize yourself with the potential pitfalls that you might face while starting out a keto diet. One way to deal with this is to keep a journal. Drinking adequate water – alone – is one of the most important things that beginners can do to avoid problems. You should keep a journal that tracks how many glasses of water you're drinking daily. That way you can precisely plan how to proceed if you're showing symptoms like dry mouth or headaches that could indicate inadequate water intake.

You can use your journal or diary for other purposes too, such as tracking the amount of protein and carbohydrate consumed each day. By writing down everything, you eat it will be easy to pinpoint problem areas.

Our next tip is don't wait for problems to arise. Make sure you have important supplements in hand before you go full blown with a ketogenic diet. Magnesium may be a vital supplement you need to get a good brand of 250 mg or 500 mg magnesium supplements to have on hand in case you start showing symptoms of problems. In fact, that level of magnesium dosage is virtually harmless while providing many benefits, so it wouldn't hurt to simply add at least 250 mg to your diet right away. This can help keep you "regular" and avoid more concerning problems like heart palpitations.

Sleep is vital for all of us, and that's especially the case when making a major change in your life. And keto is a significant change for most people. Make sure you carve out time to get your beauty rest! And, make sure you have a comfortable mattress and don't take your smartphone to bet with you!

Get some exercise. Even if you don't feel like it because keto is making you feel low energy, moderate exercise can go a long way in helping your body overcome problems like irritability and keto flu quickly. You don't need to kill yourself either. Just add a 30-minute walk to your daily routine.

Monitor your progress. Weigh yourself frequently but not daily. Also, if you can afford to do so, buy a ketone monitor so you'll know if you're really in keto or not. There is no sense guessing when the technology to find out is readily available.

Running into a wall? How often do you hear people who are dieting that stop making progress? If you do keto right and follow it carefully, this shouldn't happen. But if it does – consider taking a day off. Just don't make it a habit. But a single day off where you eat all the carbs you want can help your body reset and over the long term, you'll lose more weight. Don't let it become a trap. However, the idea of a day off might turn into two days off, then three or more if you're not a disciplined personality type. Limit yourself to a maximum of two days off per month.

Chapter 2: Starting the Ketogenic Diet

Now you have an idea of what the keto diet is all about, what ketogenesis is and what the pitfalls are. It's time to get started!

How to Start a Keto Diet

The first step in starting a diet is to compile a food list. It's quite simple to get started. The first thing is to note your protein limit. It's good to keep a notebook, so you don't stray outside your boundaries and run into roadblocks.

The general rule of thumb is to keep protein consumption to 0.45-0.5 grams of protein per pound of body weight per day. So, if you weigh 160 pounds, the amount of protein you should eat per day is 80 grams. That's a fair amount of protein. On the inside of your notebook write down your starting weight and a few reminders, like the protein limit per day and a list of prohibited foods.

Now that you know how much protein you can eat per day, what sources of protein are allowed? Virtually everything!

- All animal protein is allowed. Just make sure you're observing your daily protein limit.

- All seafood is allowed. You'll want to seek out high-fat fish, like salmon, swordfish, tuna, mackerel, and sardines. You can eat lean seafood as well but watch that protein count and be sure to pair it with other high-fat food items like avocado.

- In the early stages at least, avoid nuts. Avoid fruits and berries at all cost.

- No bread, wheat, pasta, rice, or potatoes. That includes sweet potatoes.

- Eat leafy green vegetables, cauliflower, and broccoli. But remember they do contain some carbs so don't eat unlimited amounts.

- Avoid tomatoes, at least for the first couple of months.

- Try using coconut oil and coconut cream, good sources of MCT fats.

- Avocados are an excellent addition to a ketogenic diet. An avocado is a fruit but very low in carbs and high in fat. Also provides many essential vitamins and minerals.

Who Benefits the Most from a Ketogenic Diet?

Who benefits from the keto diet? Anyone who wants to lose weight! But certain people in particular, will really excel on the keto diet. The first group of people is those who simply end up starting a diet like Atkins and then hitting a wall. If you try a diet like that and you start losing weight but find yourself stagnant or even gaining weight back a couple of weeks later, then keto might be a better option for you. You will benefit from the keto diet because it keeps proteins in check better than Atkins, South Beach, and the paleo diet.

People will slow metabolisms (that don't have documented thyroid problems) will benefit from keto. It's possible your slow metabolism is a result of problems with digesting and processing carbohydrates.

Prediabetics are probably the number one group of people that benefit on the keto diet. If you haven't been diagnosed with diabetes yet but tend to have high fasting blood sugars and you're gaining weight around your midsection but don't have any other serious health problems, then the keto diet is definitely one you will benefit from. The keto diet will normalize your blood sugars, help you lose weight fast and correct other metabolic problems often associated with prediabetes.

Type 2 diabetics can also benefit from the keto diet. But go over the possible risks that we discussed in the previous chapter, and always be sure to consult the ketogenic diet with your doctor before starting it.

Finally, let's note that both men and women benefit from the keto diet. If you need to lose weight, it doesn't matter what your gender is.

Avoiding Common Beginner's Mistakes

To avoid common beginner mistakes, the first advice is to track your activities, at least for the first couple of weeks. Some tips are:

- Drink adequate amounts of water. Use your intuition to know if you're getting enough water or not. If you find yourself having dry mouth problems, drink more.

- Make sure you're not going over your protein limits. This is the most common mistake made with keto. Remember that if you eat more than 0.5 grams of protein per pound of your body weight per day, your liver will convert some protein into blood sugar ruining the diet. Be sure to track this accurately, as you lose weight you might need to cut back on protein some more.

- Plan ahead for eating out. Don't let yourself get into a situation where "cheating" becomes necessary by eating a sandwich or slice of pizza.

- Watch for hidden carbs. Another common mistake made by beginners is to eat some fatty meat, but pile on some sugary sauces with it. Unfortunately, many favorites like barbecue sauce or teriyaki sauce can be loaded with sugar. When eating at home be sure to include the counts of carbohydrates in any sauces you use toward your total daily limit. When eating out, you can run into trouble because you may not know how many carbs are in a given sauce or salad dressing.

- Hidden carbs you may not be thinking of. You might think of cream or half and half as fatty. And they are – but they also contain carbohydrates. The amount of carbohydrates is minimal, but you need to keep track of every gram. And if you decide to consume a large amount of cream, you're going to need to know how many carbs you're dragging along. Cream is better than half-and-half, which is the watered-down version that retains the carbohydrates with less fat.

- Don't overeat fat. This advice might strike you as odd since we've been singing the praises of following a high fat diet plan! But it's true, calories still matter and you can overdo it with the fat as well. But this isn't weight watchers. You don't have to tally up points or use a calorie counter. Simply don't eat if you're not hungry – and that means fat too.

- Never really getting into ketosis. Second, to eating too much protein, this is the most serious beginner mistake. If you can afford it and you're committed to the diet, get a ketosis meter. That way you'll know you're in the Goldilocks range of 1.5-3.0 mmol/L.

- Taking too many cheat days. If you decide to approach this diet with cheat days, don't do it unless you can limit the number of cheat days to two or fewer per month and you're sure you'll stick to it. Like everything else, it's good to track your cheat days in a journal or diary so that you KNOW where you stand. This will help you avoid major mistakes like taking two, then three, and then four cheat days in a month and finding out you haven't lost any weight.

Keto Foods and How They Affect the Body

Keto foods - provided that the amount of protein they contain is within the daily limits you're allowed – help you go into ketosis! We already know what the effects of ketosis are, so it's no mystery how keto foods impact the body. Keto foods will help you burn ketones instead of glucose. As a result, they can lead to rapid weight loss and all the other practical effects of ketosis we've already discussed.

Prohibited Foods

The list of prohibited foods on keto is long, but luckily, it's very easy to follow.

- Bread: Avoid all forms of bread, including whole grains. Simply put, on keto, you aren't going to eat bread. There are some commercially available low carb bread available, but they tend to be lacking. A good rule of thumb is to avoid bread all together for the first month or two and put wheat-based bread on the do not consume list. After you've been on keto for a while, search online for low carb breads that are made from substances like almond flour. But even then, make sure you know the exact number of carbs per serving.

- Pizza. We can qualify this one. If you can make a low carb crust and eat your pizza without going over 30 grams of carbohydrate per day, then you can eat pizza. But remember it can be full of hidden carbs in many places – like tomato sauce. Be sure to count accurately. Regular pizza from a store is strictly prohibited.

- Fruit juices. People think of orange juice, or apple juice is healthy, but the reality is they are some of the worst foods you can consume. Don't drink fruit juice.

- Sodas, both diet and regular.

- Beer, in most cases.
- Root vegetables. A good rule of thumb to follow is that if a vegetable grows underground, you can't eat it. This includes carrots, turnips, potatoes, and sweet potatoes. Root vegetables are loaded with carbohydrates.

- Berries. Well actually you can consume berries, but in moderation and be sure to count the carbohydrates accurately. The best berries are the ones that are lowest in net sugar, including strawberries, blackberries, and raspberries. Blueberries are acceptable in smaller quantities, but they have more carbs than those already mentioned.

- Fruits. Think of a fruit as a natural sugar factory. Despite claims that they are necessary for health, you don't want to eat fruit on a keto diet. The lone exception is the avocado. Peaches might be one exception of a sugary fruit you can have in moderation.

- Pasta. Think of pasta like bread. Pasta is loaded with carbohydrates. A small serving would wreck your entire days' carbohydrate limits. It doesn't matter if its whole grain or not – don't eat pasta.

- Rice. Don't eat rice, even wild rice, and brown rice.

- Beans and legumes. While beans are a high protein food that is fiber-rich, they still contain too many carbohydrates for a keto diet. This is one reason why a vegetarian lifestyle isn't very compatible with keto.

- Sugar.

Beverages: What Is OK to Drink and What to Avoid

The simplest rule to follow is to drink water. However, it's possible to incorporate some other beverages into your keto lifestyle. Alcohol is a special case that we'll consider in the next chapter.

Don't drink sodas. And that means diet soda as well. You want to stay as natural as possible, and scientific research has shown that even diet sodas can cause weight gain. It's not entirely clear why that's the case, but the odds are that this type of phenomenon is going to be worse on keto. But one important aspect of soda including diet soda is how it's going to impact your fluid balance and hydration levels. We'll avoid mystery – the impacts are negative. You'll have to drink a lot of water to get back into balance after drinking a diet soda. It's best to avoid them simply.

Coffee and tea are permitted, but remember that they're diuretics. It does without saying you won't add sugar to your coffee or tea. Half and half should be avoided because although it's considered "fatty," it's watered down leaving a higher carb content. Use heavy cream instead, but don't use it in unlimited amounts. Cream has a small number of carbohydrates in it.

Something to consider is using butter in your coffee. A British cardiologist has recommended this.

Finally, avoid all "processed" drinks like red bull and other energy drinks.

Sugar and Artificial Sweeteners

Sugar is to be avoided at all costs. Calories and carbohydrates from sugar can add up quickly. If you put two teaspoons of sugar into a cup of tea, that's nearly 10 grams of carbs. If you're just starting and limiting yourself to 20 grams of carbs per day, that means you've already reached 50% of your daily limit. So, it's a good idea just to avoid it. Brown sugar is also to be avoided.

Opinions vary on artificial sweeteners. As far as safety, the reality is artificial sweeteners are safe. Any studies showing they can cause cancer have used absurd amounts. In a study that showed mice got cancer from Splenda, the mice were fed a diet equivalent to a human consuming 12,000 packs of Splenda per day. At that level, it's probably the case that anything causes cancer. Even water can kill you if you drink a massive amount over a short period.

The best advice to follow with artificial sweeteners is to consume in moderation. You can add two packs of Splenda or other artificial sweeteners to your coffee without having much impact on your diet. Just don't overdo it.

Stevia and xylitol are also acceptable options but remember to consume in moderation.

Required Ratios of Macronutrients

The key to keto is low carb, moderate protein, and high fat. But what does that mean, exactly? Let's take a look.

First, we might formally define what a "macro" is. In short macros are the general classes of nutrients as protein, fat, carbohydrate. It's also possible to include fiber and water in macros, but we won't do that here. Our focus will be on the big three: protein, fat, and carbs.

The general rule you want to follow is:

- 60-75% of calories from fat.
- 15-30% of calories from protein.
- 5-10% of calories from carbs.

You don't have to match up exactly with each meal, which is why there are allowed ranges that will let you stay in ketosis. While this information is useful, it's often easier to simply follow these rules:

- Eat a maximum of 30 grams of carbohydrate per day. Try to limit intake to 20 grams most days.
- Eat an amount of protein proportional to your body weight as we've already discussed. If you eat a half a gram of protein per pound of body weight per day, you won't have to struggle to worry about macronutrients.

Types of Fats: Good and Bad Fats

By now you've heard about bad fats. You've probably been brainwashed about bad fats nearly your entire life! The good news is that there really aren't many bad fats.

The good fats are natural, wholesome fats that include the following:

- *Monounsaturated fat.* The best sources are olive oil, avocado oil, or just eating avocados. Peanut oil is also a good fat.

- *Omega-3 oils.* These are the heart-healthy oils found in fatty fish. There are much fish you can eat on keto; the best are high-fat fish like salmon, sardines, anchovies, swordfish, and mackerel.

- *MCT oils.* The primary source of MCT fats is coconut oil. When you become more knowledgeable about the keto diet, you might be able to use MCT oils to increase your protein intake while still remaining in ketosis. Palm oils also contain MCTs and add a lot of interesting flavor to foods.

- *Saturated fats.* Yes, the devil has arrived. Doctors and nutritionists have unfairly demonized saturated fats for decades, but recent research has shown that it was all unjustified. The fact is if you're not eating a lot of carbs consuming saturated fats is just fine. Consider adding more butter to your diet.

There is only one real bad fat, and that's artificially manufactured trans-fats. This type of fat has been used for deep frying and in processed foods for decades. There is no doubt about the fact that artificial trans-fats are not good for you and raise your risk of heart disease. Of course, it's not like a molecule of the plague, one gram of trans-fats here and there is not going to send you to an early grave. But consuming them regularly can raise bad cholesterol and triglycerides while lowering your good cholesterol.

It's important to note that there are natural trans-fats. You will find these in some beef products. These should not be confused with artificially produced varieties, and there isn't any evidence that they cause health problems.

Finally, we come to vegetable oils. Some would classify them as bad fats, and if consumed in large amounts that's a fair characterization. In moderation, however, they aren't necessarily bad for you, but on a keto diet, they should be avoided. You should cook with olive oil or butter, and avoid fats like corn oil, canola oil, sunflower oil, and other similar omega-6 based oils.

The Role of Carbs in a Ketogenic Diet

Simply put when it comes to carbs you want to avoid them. The reality is the body doesn't need carbs to function; you can get by quite well on proteins and fats. However, you're going to want some carbohydrates, and in particular you're going to want those that aren't digestible. We call those kinds of carbohydrates *dietary fiber*.

An adequate amount of dietary fiber helps the body's digestive system function properly. This starts with your stomach and your small intestine and continues through the colon. A proper amount of dietary fiber will help you avoid appendicitis and helps the gall bladder perform its functions properly. Many people who are suffering from gall bladder disease may need to look at their fiber intake.

When it comes to the keto diet, two plant sources of food come to mind that are useful in not only providing needed minerals, but in providing adequate amounts of dietary fiber. The two foods we have in mind are celery and avocados. Both of these foods can be eaten in liberal quantities. Avocados, in particular, are a fantastic keto food because they are primarily a monounsaturated fat and dietary fiber. These foods will also help prevent constipation.

A second role of carbohydrates in the diet is simply as a vehicle to obtain needed antioxidants, vitamins, and minerals. Foods like spinach are packed with important minerals like potassium and magnesium, and also contain essential substances like vitamin K. Spinach contains minimal carbohydrates but does contain some, but you're not eating spinach with your steak to get energy, despite old myths. You're eating it to get the phytonutrients.

Beyond the two purposes laid out here, you don't need carbohydrates unless you have a specific health problem like type 1 diabetes. Most people can restrict their daily intake to 20 grams of carbs for very long periods – if not indefinitely – without any impact whatsoever.

Fats and proteins

When it comes to the ketogenic diet, think of fats as your energy source and proteins as a structural component. Proteins are vital for the body. People typically think of proteins as muscle – and that's one valuable role they play in the body. To avoid muscle loss with keto you'll need to be sure to get adequate protein intake as part of your diet. For most people, a protein intake of about 0.5 – 1.0 grams/pound is the right range. Don't go below 0.45 grams/pound, and always adjust your intake as you lose weight.

Keep in mind that protein isn't just about muscle mass; protein plays essential roles in the basic functioning of your body systems. For example, enzymes, which help drive the chemical reactions necessary for life, are made out of proteins. So, it's important to get adequate protein intake.

The problem with excess protein on a keto diet is that the body will use that as an excuse to make glucose. The liver can turn protein into glucose through a process known as *gluconeogenesis*. The details aren't necessary, all you need to know is that the body prefers using glucose because it's an easy energy source, and if you provide a backdoor way for the body to make glucose it's going to do it. The way that it does is by making it out of protein, and when that happens people find themselves unable to lose weight because their blood sugars are higher than they need to be.

Keeping an eye on ketones and blood sugar

Earlier we discussed a ketone meter. While it's not necessary, the best thing to do on a keto diet is to get a ketone meter and a blood glucose monitor so you know what your values are. You'll want to get baseline measurements before starting on your diet. In particular, you'll want to know your fasting blood sugar. Unless you're diabetic, it's not necessary to track your blood sugar daily, but once a week measurement to track your progress is a good idea. If you're starting with elevated blood sugars, obviously you'll want to know if keto is helping to get your blood sugar levels under control.

As we discussed earlier, you'll use a ketone meter to find out if you're actually in ketosis and how well it's going for you. Check to see if you're in the 1.5 mmol/l to 3.0 mmol/L range. If not, then take a look at what you ate that day and see if there are adjustments to be made.

As always, keep a journal or record of your numbers so you can accurately track your progress.

Best Times to Eat

Americans tend to make two major mistakes when it comes to eating no matter what kind of diet you're on. The first is skipping breakfast. We all get in a rush but skipping breakfast is a bad idea generally.

The second error people make is eating a large meal late at night. Does it make sense to consume a lot of calories and then watch TV for a while and go to sleep? It makes more sense to consume the bulk of your calories when you're more active.

Eating your big meal earlier in the day is better. In Mediterranean cultures, the big meal of the day is consumed between 1 PM – 3 PM. Consider eating a larger meal earlier in the day at lunchtime and then enjoying a smaller dinner.

This isn't strictly necessary of course, and many people are simply too busy to prepare and eat a large meal at lunch. Many don't have time to eat a large meal at lunch. However, if you're going to eat your largest meal at night, its best to eat it earlier in the evening rather than later, and you'll want to avoid eating a large meal close to bedtime.

There are options available for keto dieters who are pressed for time. Go on Amazon or to a local health food store and look for keto drink mixer options. There are many excellent mixes made for keto shakes that you can use. Some are quite tasty and satisfying, being made out of interesting foods like dried and powdered butter. Be sure to check the details and ensure that the shake is really keto friendly. Do this by checking the macronutrients. You may also consider what the shake is made out of including the protein source. Some will want whey protein, but others might prefer avoiding it.

You'll also want to give some thought about what kind of liquid you'll use if you decide to make shakes. Make sure you avoid carbs. Almond milk can be used as long as it's unsweetened. Don't use regular milk, even whole milk because it contains a large amount of carbohydrate.

Heavy cream can be used in place of milk for those looking for a high-calorie drink, but keep in mind that cream contains some carbohydrates. A cup of heavy cream contains nearly 7 grams of carbohydrate, so must be included when adding up your daily carbs. A cup of cream also contains 800 calories. While we don't count calories on keto, you do need to have some idea about it and don't want to go overboard.

Another suggestion is to mix a heavy fat like cream or even olive oil with unsweetened almond milk in your shake.

Customizing Keto

The keto diet isn't a rigid set of rules as long as you stay within the limits of ketosis. Some people will find that they can add more carbohydrates to their diet and still remain in keto, while others will have to take an approach that keeps carbs within very strict limits.

To make things interesting, you might look at other diets and find out if they can be turned into keto diets. One way to customize a keto diet is to only eat fish as your meat source, something that may work out for some.

Chapter 3: Keto and Weight Loss

We've discussed many of the benefits of a keto diet. Since the body uses ketones for fuel, the fat burning effect leads to weight loss. In many people, the weight loss will be fast and dramatic. At the beginning of the diet your body will burn a lot of glycogen, which is a form of the stored body in your muscle cells. The exciting thing about glycogen is that one glycogen molecule is bound to four water molecules. You may have heard that people on Atkins or keto lose a lot of "water weight." This is the reason that happens – your body burns up excess glycogen when faced with a new shortage of carbohydrate, and the water comes out with it. After this initial phase true and regular fat burning can begin. In this early phase, your body may go through unpleasant effects like the "keto flu" discussed earlier, but if you stick to it through this phase and make adjustments such as drinking the right amount of water and taking the right supplements, your body will adjust to such perceived maladies.

Generally speaking, people who have more body fat are going to do better on keto than people who start with relatively less weight to lose.

After the initial adjustment phase, your body is now used to being on keto. During this phase, you'll find you have better energy and mental clarity. Weight loss will be more gradual during this phase, but if you stay in ketosis, you can expect to continue losing a couple of pounds per week.

A ketogenic diet is going to be the most effective if you're one of those people who have trouble with carbohydrates. You don't have to be a diabetic either. Keto is going to result in massive weight loss for anyone who's been eating the standard American diet and steadily gaining weight over the years. But the fact is millions of people are literally being poisoned by having too many carbohydrates in their diet and aren't even aware of it.

Even if diabetes isn't something in your genes, the more you pile on the carbs in your diet the harder you're making your pancreas work. The body's cells become insulin resistant, meaning that they're less responsive to a given amount of insulin in the bloodstream. The result? More insulin is required to accomplish the same amount of work. For some people over time no amount of insulin gets the job done − those are the people who have diabetes or suffering from pre-diabetes. Other people still won't be pre-diabetes yet, but their cells are still forcing the pancreas to pump out more insulin to overcome the slowly increasing resistance. Over time this leads to more body fat, since one of the functions of insulin is to direct the body to store excess calories as body fat.

When you follow a keto lifestyle, this vicious cycle is eliminated. Instead of your body constantly battling excess sugars, it's burning fat for fuel instead. That means it will burn off your body fat and you'll start losing weight.

The biggest key with keto is people usually lose weight effortlessly. A dieter will find themselves eating fatty rib eye steaks, chicken with the skin on, avocadoes, and butter, and yet tipping the scale a little less each day. The results can come in shockingly rapid fashion. In this video, Jordan Peterson describes his weight loss − seven pounds a month for seven months in a row.

https://youtu.be/tw8Rf9ho-Sk

Most people will find they lose weight rapidly if they strictly follow a keto diet. And even those who only diet intermittently will also find they lose weight. However, you should make sure you follow the keto style of eating at least 3-4 days per week if you decide to go down that path.

Remember we said there were two caveats. The second caveat is to avoid eating too much protein. Failing to follow this rule sinks a lot of keto dieters. If you find yourself losing a lot of weight initially but then hit a plateau, consider your protein intake.

Chapter 4: Lowering Your Triglycerides

Triglycerides are a type of fat found in the blood, which are made every time you eat. While insulin will trigger the cells to take up the blood sugar they need for energy, any excess calories that have been consumed will be converted into triglycerides by the liver. Triglycerides are released into the bloodstream and then transported through the bloodstream. Triglycerides are then converted into stored fat on the body. Some people have defective liver metabolism and will produce more triglycerides than others given the same caloric and carb intake.

The biggest culprits when it comes to triglycerides are sugar and alcohol. If you consume alcohol to excess, you're probably going to raise your triglyceride levels. In fact, a problem alcoholics sometimes encounter is they increase their triglyceride levels to extremely high standards, triggering a life-threatening condition known as pancreatitis. The details aren't important here, but what happens is the pancreas works extra hard as a result of the high blood levels of triglycerides.

Fasting blood levels of triglycerides can be summarized by these categories:

- Very high: to reach this level your fasting triglyceride level would be 500 mg/dL or higher.
- High: this range is 200 to 499 mg/dL.
- Borderline: 150 to 199 mg/dL.
- Normal: Below 150 mg/dL.
- Ideal: Below 80 mg/dL.

If your triglyceride level (fasting) is borderline, your doctor is likely to advise limiting alcohol consumption and making dietary and exercise changes. Losing weight can also help lower fasting triglyceride numbers, although in some cases the cause is simple genetics or family history. If your fasting triglyceride number is high or very high, medication is likely to be prescribed.

Even if you're not an alcoholic, high triglyceride levels can put your body at risk for pancreatitis and other problems. Medical professionals consider a fasting triglyceride level of 150 or lower to be reasonable. A level below 100 is better, and 70 or below is ideal. If your fasting triglyceride level is above 200, your doctor may put you on a medication called gemfibrozil. Alternatively, triglyceride levels can be lowered with high consumption of EPA, a type of fish oil. Following this approach requires consuming at least 3,000 mg of EPA per day. While there is a prescription medication available that contains EPA, you can purchase purified EPA over the counter as well. If you decide to do so, you should make sure that you can readily get the required 3,000 mg per day of fish oil from the product. Also, be sure to consult with your doctor before consuming that much fish oil to make sure you don't have any pre-existing health problems that could lead to difficulties.

Pancreatitis isn't the only risk of high triglyceride levels. In fact, if you're not an alcoholic pancreatitis is relatively rare, except cases where the patient has bile duct problems. The main concern with high triglyceride levels is with heart disease.

We've discussed this earlier in the book. The primary dietary culprit besides alcohol consumption in high triglyceride numbers is the consumption of carbohydrates, in particular simple sugars. Many doctors will advise consuming "whole grains," but the reality is for lots of people whole gains will keep triglyceride levels elevated. Since triglyceride levels are directly related to the consumption of excess calories, it's easy to see why eating a lot of carbohydrates can raise triglyceride levels.

Your levels of triglycerides and HDL or "good" cholesterol are tied closely together. HDL means *high-density lipoprotein*. It's a type of cholesterol that actually cleans out the LDL or "bad" cholesterol from your arteries.

High triglycerides can lead to the development of heart disease. In fact, it's slowly being recognized as one of the most important factors. Type 2 diabetics in particular – and those not yet diabetic but potentially diabetic – tend to have high triglycerides. In short:

- High blood sugar levels often correspond to higher triglyceride levels and lower levels of HDL or "good" cholesterol.
- People with weight problems tend to have higher triglyceride levels.
- High triglyceride levels correspond to smaller, and denser LDL or "bad" cholesterol molecules.

Since triglycerides are transported through the bloodstream by LDL cholesterol, the fact that the body has a certain level of cholesterol it needs to transport using LDL means that crowding out by triglycerides translates into more LDL particles. Since triglycerides pack densely, this also means the particles are smaller, and so pose a greater risk of sticking to arterial walls, leading to heart disease.

Factors that influence triglyceride level include:

- Weight gain
- High fasting blood sugar levels
- More body fat
- Consumption of carbohydrates
- Alcohol
- High fasting blood sugars
- Lack of exercise

Of the factors on the list, exercise is the least important, and studies showing that exercise helps triglyceride levels might be since people who exercise are in better shape in general, having less body fat, healthier body weight, and lower blood sugar levels.

Lower HDL levels which are associated with high triglyceride and high blood sugar levels, cause problems as well. HDL or "good" cholesterol acts as a type of vacuum cleaner in the bloodstream, sucking up excess LDL molecules for transport back to the liver. By reducing LDL particle number, HDL reduces the probability that LDL molecules will stick to the arterial walls leading to heart disease. Low HDL values indicate you don't have enough HDL in your bloodstream to effectively "clean it out."

Factors that can increase HDL include:

- Losing weight.
- Exercise.
- Consumption of healthy fats like monounsaturated fats and omega-3 oils.
- Consumption of MCT fats, which are found in coconut and palm oil (be aware that coconut and palm oil also have high concentrations of saturated fats as well).

- Eating a low carbohydrate diet.

Since a ketogenic diet hits several of these points, dieters typically see their HDL increase.

We've seen that HDL level, blood sugar level, and triglyceride level are all related, but what's the connection? It turns out its insulin sensitivity. A good indirect way to measure insulin sensitivity is to check your triglyceride to HDL level. This is also a good measure of heart attack risk, as we've discussed previously. To calculate this level, you only need two pieces of data:

- Your fasting triglyceride number
- Your fasting HDL number

Then divide the triglyceride number by your HDL number. For example, suppose that Susan has a fasting triglyceride number of 180 mg/DL, and her fasting HDL value is 40 mg/dL. Then her triglyceride to HDL ratio is:

Ratio = triglycerides/HDL = 180/40 = 4.5

Any value above 3 is considered a high risk for heart disease. It also indicates that Susan has problems with insulin sensitivity, and her blood sugar is likely to be high as well. Note again that we are talking about fasting values. Note that when taken alone, even though Susan's HDL number might be considered low normal and her triglyceride level is only moderately elevated, when taken together these numbers tell us that Susan is in fact at *high risk* of heart disease. A ketogenic diet can definitely help someone like Susan, by lowering her triglyceride levels and possibly raising her HDL levels as well.

When you are insulin resistant, this means that you're producing enough insulin, but the cells are not responding properly and removing glucose from the blood. People who are insulin resistant are at higher risk of developing diabetes and may suffer from a condition called metabolic syndrome. In contrast, consider John, who has a fasting triglyceride level of 100 mg/dL and a fasting HDL value of 50 mg/dL. For John, we find a triglyceride to HDL level of:

Ratio = triglycerides/HDL = 100/50 = 2

His level is well below 3, so we consider John to be in a healthy range. He is considered at moderate risk for cardiovascular disease. However, even John could benefit from adopting a keto or low-carb diet because he could lower his triglyceride level even more. Consuming more fish can also help.

Even though the keto diet can massively improve your blood lipid numbers, it's important to exercise as well. In several large studies, it has been shown that moderate to vigorous physical activity significantly reduces the incidence of cardiovascular events such as heart attack and stroke. This has also been studied by comparing triglyceride to HDL ratios with the level of cardiovascular fitness. It has been found that levels of cardiovascular fitness and triglyceride to HDL ratios are *independent* predictors of future heart attack and stroke. Therefore, it's important to incorporate some exercise into your keto lifestyle and not rely entirely on the diet alone. It's not necessary to become a triathlete to get the benefits. You can achieve a healthy level of fitness by incorporating moderate exercise such as a daily 30-minute walk into your routine. Depending on your health status more may be required. Generally, 150 minutes of walking per week is considered to be the required level of moderate activity that will reduce cardiovascular risk. If you are engaging in more vigorous exercise, such as jogging or bicycling, the time required is lower. It's generally accepted that about half the weekly effort is necessary when pursuing vigorous exercise, so those doing so should shoot for about 75 minutes per week of activity.

Chapter 5: Normalize Your Blood Sugar

By now you've probably figured out that several risk factors for heart disease go hand-in-hand. This is known as "risk factor clustering." The risk factors for the development of heart disease that often come together in the same individuals includes (fasting values):

- Low HDL cholesterol
- High triglyceride levels
- High blood sugar levels (often high enough to be diagnosed with pre-diabetes)
- Obesity
- Low insulin sensitivity
- High blood pressure

When a person has all of these risk factors, it's called metabolic syndrome. The focal point of all of these problems tends to be high blood sugar – something that is the result of *low insulin sensitivity*.

The Impact of Keto on Insulin

A keto diet has positive impacts on insulin. Low carbohydrate consumption translates to lower levels of insulin in the body because more insulin isn't necessary. Even when not eating, the effects are felt. Keto dieters have lower levels of fasting insulin than do people that consume carbohydrates. Simply put when you have less sugar to deal with your body makes less insulin. A keto diet will lower fasting insulin levels, stabilize blood sugar, and improve insulin sensitivity. What this means is that when the body does need to use insulin, it will work more efficiently.

You can try to address insulin sensitivity by taking medications such as metformin, or you can address it naturally by changing your diet. Keto diet helps address insulin sensitivity by reducing the number of carbohydrates consumed. A natural extension of this is that fasting blood sugar levels are naturally reduced leading to a healthier overall state of the body.

A beginner's mistake often made on ketogenic diets is that people starting the ketogenic diet aren't really eating keto. This happens when people eat too much protein. When excess amounts of protein are consumed, if there are not also a lot of carbohydrates in the diet your liver will make glucose out of the protein. For this reason, it's important to maintain an adequate but moderate level of protein in your daily diet. This is done by keeping protein consumption at a level of 0.45 to 0.5 grams per pound of body weight.

For example, when Steve starts his ketogenic diet, he weighs 200 pounds. So he should consume:

- At least 90 grams of protein per day. We arrive at this number using 0.45 grams/pound * 200 pounds = 90 grams of protein.
- At most 100 grams of protein per day. We arrive at this number using 0.5 grams/pound * 200 pounds = 100 grams of protein.

It's just as important to consume an adequate amount of protein as it is to avoid consuming excess protein. If you fail to consume enough protein, then you might find yourself losing muscle tissue and not just fat. We certainly don't want to lose weight by losing muscle mass.

When Steve loses some weight, he will need to reduce his protein consumption. Let's suppose that after a week Steve has lost ten pounds. Now he weighs 190 pounds and he should adjust his protein consumption accordingly:

- At least 85.5 grams of protein per day. We arrive at this number using 0.45 grams/pound * 190 pounds = 85.5 grams of protein.
- At most 95 grams of protein per day. We arrive at this number using 0.45 grams/pound * 190 pounds = 95 grams of protein.

The takeaways are that burning ketones instead of sugar will result in lower fasting blood sugars and help deal with metabolic syndrome. By consuming the right level of proteins we ensure that we won't have hidden sources of blood sugar in our diets.

Chapter 6: Alcohol and Keto

The consumption of alcohol is something that has to be carefully considered while on the keto diet. Many people aren't aware of this, but when you're on keto and making your liver work by turning fats into usable ketone bodies, it's going to be harder for your liver to process alcohol too. That means that some people are going to have a hard time drinking while they are in ketosis. You might find yourself getting intoxicated after consuming a much smaller amount of alcohol than you're used to.

If you run into this sort of problem, you'll want to step back and figure out if drinking alcohol is all that important to you. If you decide that you want to keep drinking, you'll have to adjust your behavior accordingly. This means determining what your new limits are and even considering going off ketosis before drinking, as long as that's not a frequent occurrence. If it's something you're going to do just once in a while, you can consume a small meal of a carbohydrate-rich food before drinking alcohol. Doing so will get the liver off the hook when dealing with ketones so it will be freed up to deal with the onslaught of alcohol.

Alcohol can be consumed in moderation, but drinking too much can cause problems when it comes to losing weight, even on keto. The body will burn alcohol before it burns other fuels, so if you drink too much in one sitting, you'll find yourself not losing weight as expected. The best thing to do if you decide to drink while on keto is to follow the general advice on drinking in moderation. Using wine as an example, stick to 1-2 glasses per day for women and 2-3 glasses per day with men. Also, be aware that you'll have to know how many carbs are in the alcohol you're drinking and include it in your daily totals.

Types of alcohol that should be avoided include beer and sugary mixed drinks. Hard liquor and other spirits, as well as wine and champagne, make better options for keto dieters.

Once you've determined your limits, the next thing to do is familiarize yourself with the carb content of alcoholic drinks to determine which ones are suitable to use with keto. Let's start with the most frequently consumed drinks, beer, and wine. Obviously, details vary, but we'll use average carb loads per serving:

- Beer: 10-13 carbs (per 12 oz. serving).
- Red wine: 2 carbs (standard wine glass, 5 oz.).
- White wine: 2 carbs (standard wine glass, 5 oz.).
- Champagne: 1-2 carbs (5 oz. serving).

Be aware that sweeter tasting wines will have higher carbohydrate levels than those cited here. A typical sweet wine such as a Riesling will contain twice as many carbs or about 4 per glass. Dry wines are preferred on a keto diet.

An interesting aside is that wine is a nutritious drink. One glass of merlot, for example, contains 187 mg of potassium, 5% of the recommended daily allowance of vitamin B-6, and 4% of the recommended daily allowance of magnesium. Of course, it's not a good idea to be drinking wine to get your potassium, but it's good to know that you're getting more out of it than alcohol.

Beer is another story. If you're on a ketogenic diet, then beer is something you'll want to avoid. People tend to think of beer as starchy, and that's an accurate perception, as is the term "beer belly." It's pretty clear that if you're on a keto diet and limiting your daily carb intake to 20-30 grams per day, a "couple of beers" are going to wreck your diet totally.

Craft beers and varieties like IPA are even worse. A 12-ounce Sierra Nevada IPA contains 175 calories and 14 grams of carbs. Many IPAs have even more carbs, some up to 20 grams per serving. Making things even worse is the fact that if you go out somewhere, chances are you're not going to be getting a 12-ounce serving. Most places will serve beer in pints or 22-ounce sizes. This means that drinking beer adds a lot of carbohydrates to your daily intake.

Hard drinks or so-called "spirits" offer low or zero carb options. Soda water (unsweetened) can be used to make a low carb mixed drink. Some *zero* carb options include:

- Whiskey
- Tequila
- Vodka
- Dry martini
- Brandy

Mixed drinks are more problematic and need to be chosen with care. Many contain sugary syrups and carbohydrates as the main ingredient. A margarita contains 8 carbs per serving while a white Russian contains around 17. A bloody Mary checks in at around 7 carbs per serving. Adding orange juice or sugary sodas to your drink can create a high sugar drink with a large number of carbs double or more these values, so it's probably best to avoid them. Mixed drinks that only use carbonated sodas and lime or lemon (for example) are usually low carb and make good substitutes.

Chapter 7: Cholesterol and Keto

One of the major objections raised with keto is that it will raise your cholesterol. For many people it will raise it, but it's important to look at the details. Doctors used to look only at the total cholesterol number, but have since discovered there are different types and subtypes of cholesterol. When it comes to keto, it's important to understand what they are and know their values to make sense out of your numbers.

Cholesterol is basically a kind of fatty material. Since fat and water don't mix, the body packages cholesterol with a type of protein so that it can be transported through the blood. The bound molecules are called a *lipoprotein*, meaning fat + protein. The proteins that are a part of cholesterol help move it through the blood to where it needs to go in the body. Cholesterol is a very useful substance, it's used to help build cell membranes and to manufacture important hormones in the body like vitamin-d and testosterone. People who have very low levels of "bad" cholesterol are actually at higher risk of death from all causes. Your body needs "bad" cholesterol, you don't want too much and having it stick to the walls of your arteries, clogging up the pipes and doing damage.

By now everyone has heard about *good* and *bad* cholesterol. Good cholesterol is called HDL. HDL means "high-density lipoprotein," and it's called "good" cholesterol because its function in the body is to remove the LDL or "bad" cholesterol from your bloodstream. This helps protect against the buildup of plaque in your arteries.

A high HDL number means a lower long-term risk of heart disease. For most people, following a keto lifestyle will raise your HDL number. It turns out that several blood markers – HDL, triglycerides, and blood sugar – tend to be related in how they move in response to diet. While not true in all cases, for most people weight gain and problems maintaining healthy blood sugar levels correspond to lower HDL numbers and higher triglyceride numbers. This is fixed by going into ketosis, and the best way to do that is to eat a ketogenic diet. To summarize:

A higher HDL number means a lower risk of heart disease, and most people will see their HDL number go up while following a keto diet.

LDL stands for low-density lipoprotein, and it's known as "bad" cholesterol because more LDL translates into a higher risk of heart disease – generally speaking. When doctors talk about high cholesterol numbers, they are talking about the LDL number, and most blood tests now give a specific measurement for LDL.

However, it turns out that just knowing your LDL number doesn't tell the whole story. The size of LDL particles is also important. Smaller LDL particles are more likely to stick to your artery walls and cause cardiovascular disease. A ketogenic diet will make LDL particles larger, while a diet high in carbohydrates tends to make them smaller.

- A ketogenic diet makes LDL or "bad" cholesterol molecules light and fluffy. They can travel through the blood stream without doing much damage.
- A diet high in carbohydrates, especially a sugar-laden diet, will make LDL particles small and hard, making them more likely to stick to artery walls and cause cardiovascular disease.

These two facts explain a lot. In particular, it describes why saturated fat has been associated with heart disease in the past. Saturated fat is made into LDL cholesterol by the liver. So eating more saturated fat from beef or chicken skin can raise your LDL number. Now we see where the confusion comes in. If you're eating a lot of saturated fat *and* following a high carbohydrate diet, your LDL number will go up, and the LDL particles will be hard, small, and sticky – leading to heart disease.

However, if you are following a low carb diet, especially a keto diet, the saturated fat you consume is going to be packaged by the liver into light and fluffy LDL particles that travel through the blood stream without sticking to your arterial walls and causing heart disease. You can summarize this by saying it's not the beef patty that causes heart disease in the typical American diet, it's *the beef patty together with the French fries and bun* that cause heart disease.

- A diet that is high in carbohydrates should limit saturated fat to keep LDL cholesterol lower. The combination of saturated fat + carbohydrates tends to produce smaller and dangerous LDL particles. Doctors typically recommend limiting saturated fat to 20 grams or less if you are eating a normal diet with a high number of carbohydrates.
- A diet that is low in carbohydrates can be high in saturated fat because the LDL particles will be light and fluffy, and heart disease does not develop. On the keto diet you can eat saturated fat without worrying about it.

Now we learn that triglycerides play a role here too. LDL particles carry triglycerides with them, and the more triglycerides they carry the fewer cholesterol molecules they carry. Think of it as an airplane with a fixed number of seats, and people are wearing green suits or white suits. Let's also suppose that the people in green suits were going on optional flights, but the people in white suits were going on required flights.

The more people are wearing green suits (triglycerides) that board the plane, the fewer people wearing white suits (cholesterol) that can board the plane. So to transport all the people in white suits to their destinations, the more airplanes you need. On the other hand, if there were fewer people in green suits, more people with white suits could board the airplane and you'd have fewer airplanes and fewer flights.

That is one reason why high triglycerides raise the risk of heart disease. They take up space in your LDL particles, and so the body needs more LDL particles to transport cholesterol. It also affects the density of the LDL particles. You can think of them as small and hard. Small and hard LDL particles stick to artery walls and cause heart disease.

Conversely, if you have lower levels of triglycerides, there is more room for cholesterol in an LDL particle. So a given LDL particle packs more cholesterol in it, and it's going to be larger in size, light and fluffy. LDL particles that are light and fluffy don't stick to artery walls and don't raise heart disease risk.

These observations explain a lot, including why a keto diet is healthy and effective. One of the most important effects of the keto diet is to lower triglycerides. So while an increased consumption of fats, saturated fat in particular, may raise total cholesterol in some people and total LDL cholesterol, it does not mean your heart disease risk has increased. You can have your doctor track your LDL-P number (where P is for particle number) as well as the LDL number, so you can learn how your particle number is progressing. A higher cholesterol number with a lower LDL-P means you're in a healthier state. So let's summarize the impact of keto on cholesterol:

- Following a keto diet lowers triglycerides.
- A keto diet tends to increase HDL.
- More HDL means that LDL or bad cholesterol is cleaned out from the bloodstream more effectively; lowering the risk you'll develop plaque.
- A lower triglyceride number means that you'll have fewer LDL particles, each of which carries more cholesterol per particle. They will be larger, and "fluffy" and not stick to arterial walls, so don't raise the risk of heart disease.

If you're not able to get a detailed LDL profile with your blood lipid tests, you can simply use triglycerides as a proxy. A level below 150 is the standard value considered healthy by the medical establishment. Many on a keto diet will see their triglyceride level drop below 100 and even into the range of 50-60.

Finally, remember to track your triglyceride to HDL value. Get your triglyceride number and divide it by the HDL number to get the ratio.

- If your triglyceride to HDL ratio is 3 or more, you're at higher risk of heart disease.
- If your triglyceride to HDL ratio is less than 3, you're at decreased risk of heart disease.

As discussed above, the keto diet is likely to cause the following changes to your cholesterol panel:

- Your HDL cholesterol will rise.

- Your LDL cholesterol may rise, causing total cholesterol to rise.
- However, your LDL-P number will decrease, indicating better health.
- Your triglyceride levels will decrease.

Why High Total Cholesterol Isn't Necessarily Bad

As discussed above, high total cholesterol isn't necessarily bad. When you go on a keto diet your triglyceride levels will decrease, and HDL may increase. So, if you're total cholesterol an increase, this likely reflects that your HDL level has increased. Moreover, your LDL level has probably increased as well, but the type of LDL molecules is more important than the raw number. If possible, find out how your LDL-P number is changing with time. A keto diet likely means that you're going to have larger and less damaging LDL particles and there will be fewer in number, even though the raw cholesterol number may be higher. The best metric you should keep track of is the triglyceride to HDL value. A lower value indicates a healthier LDL.

Earlier we discussed a ketone meter, it's also possible to buy a home meter that checks your cholesterol, HDL, and triglyceride levels. You will have to infer your overall LDL cholesterol number as this test is not available with existing home meters. An excellent meter to look at is called *Cardiochek*. You can find out your triglyceride and HDL numbers and track your ratios. Be sure to only test fasting values, and go 8-12 hours without eating before doing the test. The device is FDA approved, but you may want to repeat tests and average because the error rate will be higher than that seen with a test done at the doctor's office, with a larger amount of blood.

Chapter 8: Incorporating Exercise into a Keto Lifestyle

The main issue with exercise and keto is that at first, your body enters a transition period where you might experience low energy levels and brain "fog." Deprived of glucose, your body has to adjust to making and using ketone bodies for energy. For some people this is not a problem, while others will have to adjust to the "keto flu." The good news is that this will pass once your body becomes fully adjusted and your energy levels will increase.

If you suffer from this issue, you shouldn't stop exercising, but you probably won't want to hit it hard or add new challenges to your exercise routine either. The key to exercise and keto is consuming enough fat.

Once you transition to keto fat is your energy source, so it's important that you genuinely consume the levels of fat the diet demands. If you eat enough fat, then you'll have enough energy for your workouts and find that you burn more fat off your body when you do exercise.

Some recent research into the benefits of exercise has uncovered surprises that might be to the liking of most readers. Previously, it had been thought that to attain cardiovascular fitness a person had to engage in 20 or 30 minutes of "vigorous" exercise per day to get the benefits. When researchers studied people who were regular runners, however, they came across a stunning result – people who only ran five minutes a day got most of the health benefits that those running 30 minutes or an hour got from their running. The runners were followed over a long time period, and it was found that all runners had a lower risk of death and cardiovascular disease as compared to people who didn't exercise, or did so at moderate levels. But the differences between those who ran only five minutes and those running for long time periods wasn't really all that significant. You can find a nice lay person's discussion of this research in the New York Times.

So it appears that people get the majority of the benefit that hard cardiovascular training provides after only a short period of exercising.

This surprising result provides an alternative for people who aren't very excited about putting in long days at the gym. It may be possible that you can get the same benefits by just going on a short jog.

Now we aren't giving out specific health advice in this book, so it's up to each individual to do the research and find out what works best for him or her. One possible way to rev up your exercise without having to kill yourself is to do a 30-minute walk three or four days a week, and do a five-minute jog three days a week. That way you're getting a little bit of both.

At the time of writing, researchers aren't sure if the five-minute benefits accrue to other types of exercise. So they aren't sure if riding on an exercise bike for five minutes a day will provide the same benefits or not, but common sense seems to imply that it would if you use a good level of intensity.

In any case, when it comes down to exercise, you need to tailor it both to your own needs and also to something you like doing. Enjoyment of exercise is directly proportional to how much you do and whether or not you stick to it.

It's important to note that on a keto lifestyle, exercise is not strictly required. Simply following a keto diet will enable you to lose weight and do so rapidly and consistently, provided that you're strictly following the guidelines. However, for optimal health cardiovascular exercise is recommended. In large-scale studies that have tracked people for blood markers like triglycerides, HDL cholesterol, and total cholesterol, as well as tracking their exercise habits, it has been found that those who exercised and managed their blood lipids were at the lowest risk of heart attack and stroke.

Those who exercised but didn't maintain good blood lipids had lower cardiovascular risk than people who didn't exercise at all, but had higher cardiovascular risk than people who exercised and had good blood lipids. Conversely, those who had good blood lipid profiles had lower cardiovascular risk than the general population. However, if they didn't exercise, they had a higher risk than those who exercised and had good blood lipids.

What are we saying here? The bottom line is that having good blood lipids, as defined by low triglycerides, low LDL or "bad" cholesterol, and high HDL, as well as low blood sugar is very important. And you'll get this profile by following a keto diet carefully.

However, people who do this *and* exercise are at the lowest risk.

The goal of exercising should be to obtain a minimal level of cardiovascular fitness. It's not the time spent exercising or what you do that appears to be important, but whether you've conditioned your body in such a way that you can withstand the challenge that says a five-minute run entails.

If you don't exercise at all, a five-minute run might be extremely challenging. Many middle-aged or older people who don't engage in regular exercise will be able to run *even that much*. That's why a five-minute jog is probably connected to significantly lower risks of heart attack and stroke – because that small amount of time commitment is enough to condition the body.

Believe it or not, some recent research has taken this concept even further. Some researchers have found that a one or two minutes of aerobic exercise appears to condition people's bodies well enough that cardiovascular disease risk is significantly reduced. What we're talking about here is running all-out sprints for at least one minute, as hard and fast as you can run.

Exercising just a minute a day might sound very appealing – and it might work out for you. But, If you have an underlying heart problem and run at an all-out sprint, it might be enough to trigger a heart attack.

We should also mention that cardiovascular disease isn't the only risk factor that short bouts of exercise appear to impact. They also appear to reduce the risk of death from all causes.

Chapter 9: Keto and Insomnia

Lack of sleep is a significant health problem, leading to obesity, overeating, hormone changes and other health problems. If you don't get good nights sleep, you'll have trouble making it through the day and mentally focusing.

For some people, keto may cause insomnia problems in the early stages of the diet. In most cases, this is driven by the "keto flu." The odds are that it will pass once your body fully adjusts and you're burning ketones for fuel. The key here is the same as it is with exercise – make sure you're getting enough fat in your diet. If you're feeling low energy and not getting good nights sleep, consider increasing your fat intake.

Conversely, you might be getting more energy from fat. That is keto is working out really well for you, but you're so energetic that going to sleep is more difficult. In that case, try eating your last meal earlier in the evening.

Another problem that causes insomnia on keto is depletion of your glycogen stores. Glycogen is sugar stored in your muscle cells. Each glycogen molecule is bound to four molecules of water. People who need to lose weight not only have extra fat they're carrying around, they also have higher glycogen stores on average.

When you start the keto diet one of the things that happen is your body rapidly uses up its excess storage of glycogen, to keep burning sugars for fuel. This is a good thing – you'll be healthier once you're rid of this excess. But an unpleasant side effect of this is that you'll probably be urinating more than you're used to as the body gets rid of the water that has been stored with the glycogen. This is the proverbial 'water weight' problem.

So what happens when you have to pee a lot more? You might find yourself having to go more at night, and getting up frequently to go to the bathroom can cause insomnia problems. The good news is that this problem will pass in a short period once your glycogen stores become adjusted to a reasonable level.

The final factor that can lead to insomnia problems on a keto diet is an improper electrolyte balance. We've seen this problem rear its ugly head before in other areas. So make sure that you're not just focused on fat and meat – get your minerals. Try drinking a cup of broth every day and make sure you're also getting adequate potassium and magnesium to keep your sodium in balance. You can take magnesium supplements, but great sources of potassium and magnesium include leafy greens like spinach, broccoli, and avocados, which also contain large amounts of healthful monounsaturated fat. When eaten in moderation, macadamia nuts can also help provide needed minerals and monounsaturated fats, but they shouldn't be consumed until you've been on the diet for a few weeks. Also, keep track of any carbs you consume from nuts.

Chapter 10: Keto and Acne

A surprising benefit of the keto diet is that in some people, keto will decrease and even cure acne problems. Over the past few decades, people didn't connect acne with diet because research had failed to link high levels of acne to specific foods. However, the problem was they weren't looking at macros, and during most of the research period people weren't interested in a keto diet.

It turns out that acne is related to hormonal imbalances. In your skin, sebaceous glands produce oils that keep your skin lubricated. In people with serious acne problems, this process is disrupted.

Elevated androgens cause the production of a compound called *sebum* in the skin as well as make the skin more oily. Sebum can clog skin pores, which also traps bacteria that were on your skin. A small infection results and you develop a pimple, which is simply the body's attempt to trap, isolate and get rid of an infection. In short, acne is an inflammatory response. Androgens are "male" hormones, and more of them are produced in adolescence and young adulthood, which is why teenagers are more likely to produce acne. Many adults have problems with acne as well.

And guess what can exacerbate these types of hormonal imbalances? A high level of carbohydrate consumption. Keto immediately fixes this problem and so many people on keto find that their acne has been substantially reduced.

In the early stages of the diet, however, you might find your acne worsening. You can relax about this knowing that like other effects this is likely to be temporary. People more prone to issues like keto flu may also have temporarily worsening acne. As the body adjusts to burning fat and depleting excess glycogen stores, it's also going to adjust proper hormone levels that can impact acne. If you're in this situation give it a short amount of time. Over time a keto diet – followed closely without cheating – will lead to clearer skin.

There are several reasons for this. Remember that a keto diet will result in lower insulin levels. It turns out that high insulin levels also contribute to more oils and sebum in the skin, raising the risk of acne problems. The second factor that contributes to reducing acne is that keto diets reduce inflammation overall. Remember that acne is an inflammatory response. When you have less inflammation, you're less likely to develop acne.

Finally, a special hormone called *insulin-like growth factor-1* or IGF-1 has been shown to increase the propensity to develop acne. It turns out that ketogenic diets will reduce levels of IGF-1 in the body, and therefore reduce the propensity to develop acne.

Chapter 11: Keto and Stress

It can be said that a ketogenic diet is an elixir for mental health. There have been hints of this for centuries since it was known that keto diets helped control epilepsy in children. But it has taken a long time to connect the benefits of keto to other brain functions, including mental clarity and better mental health.

High blood sugars cause stress at the cellular level and with this comes the release of stress hormones like cortisol. This causes feelings of stress and inflammation throughout the body. The result is you feel more stress and anxiety in your mental states.
By reducing carbohydrates, the level of stress at the cellular level and beyond is also reduced. Stress hormones like cortisol are released in smaller amounts, and this creates a better mental perception.

People on keto will find that they have lower rates of anxiety, sleep better, and have lower perceptions of stress overall. But keep in mind that once again, the "keto flu" phenomena might influence your early experiences on the keto diet. That means initially you might find your stress and anxiety levels increase – but like other aspects of keto flu, this is temporary.

The keto diet addresses stress and anxiety primarily by regulating hormones. High blood sugars can wreak havoc by causing stress that leads your adrenal glands to release various hormones. This problem is made worse in people that have even moderate difficulties with blood sugar, in particular with blood sugar "spikes." Even ordinary people have blood sugar spikes – if you eat a meal with a large component of carbohydrates about two hours after eating your blood sugar will spike.

In a supposedly healthy person, it might spike at 140 mmol/L. In a person with metabolic syndrome or pre-diabetes, the level may go as high as 180 mmol/L. People with diabetes might see it go much higher if they aren't being treated.

You can do a simple test at home with a blood sugar meter and some orange juice, to see how your body responds to blood sugar. Drink an 8-ounce glass of orange juice and wait two hours. Then check your blood sugar and see how high it rises. If it's higher than 140 mmol/L, then you definitely have issues with blood sugar. But again – you probably don't want it going to 140 in the first place.

Fluctuating blood sugar levels will cause fluctuating levels of stress hormones as well. This is independent of other methods used to control stress like medication. We can avoid this problem by following a keto diet. The keto diet will keep blood sugar levels confined to a narrow range. As a result, stress hormones released in response to fluctuating blood sugars will also be consistent as well, reducing overall stress on the body and keeping you healthier.

Even those with high fasting blood sugars will find that they don't experience any spikes on keto, and even before their fasting blood sugar levels improve they will see better A1C values. For example, if you are pre-diabetic and typically have a fasting blood sugar of 120, you will probably find that eating keto meals your blood sugar only bounces around between 120 and 130, rather than dropping to 100 and then spiking to 180 like it would when eating a carbohydrate-rich diet.

Try doing a second test to see how your body responds with a high fat meal. Before eating, take your blood sugar to get a baseline number. Then eat a fatty meal, with macros of fat, protein, and carbohydrates in proper proportion. Then two hours after taking your first bite retake your blood sugar and check the results. You will find that it will be very close to your baseline number, in contrast to the results you're going to see when doing the orange juice test.

Chapter 12: Keto and Intermittent Fasting

Many people like to incorporate fasting into their keto lifestyle. This can be beneficial for increasing weight loss, and we will see why in a minute. However, it's important to note that fasting is not required for a keto lifestyle. The contents of this chapter are entirely optional.

Fasting Overview

Fasting has been used since the beginning of time as a means of attaining optimal health. Surprisingly, the body may be adapted to some level of fasting. During prehistoric times, game animals and fruits and vegetables were in short supply at times. If human beings were so fragile that they required constant food consumption, they would have vanished a long time ago, and we wouldn't be here today having this conversation. If it took a few extra days to hunt down an animal to get valuable fats and proteins, then the body had to be adapted to being able to go for short periods without food.

It turns out that fasting can be good for you. As always, you should check with your doctor first before starting a fasting program. In the keto world, we call this intermittent fasting because it's something you'll do periodically but not all the time. The benefits that have been tied to fasting are numerous and include:

- Increased weight loss
- Stabilized blood sugars
- Lower blood pressure
- Longer lifespan
- Reduction and even reversal of type 2 diabetes

Diabetics, in particular, should speak to their doctor before adopting a fasting program. Intermittent fasting can have important implications for medications used to treat diabetes. Intermittent fasting also shouldn't be used if you're underweight or have other serious problems such as cancer.

However, if you're in the proper health to incorporate fasting, it's something that you'll want to consider adding to your keto lifestyle.

How Keto Can Be Correlated with Fasting

It's when we look into the details of fasting that we find its connection to the keto diet. You probably won't be surprised. After all, what happens when your body isn't getting a lot of carbohydrates that it can use for energy? Your body makes ketones. So, what happens when we're fasting, and not taking in any carbohydrates?

You guessed it – when you're fasting your body makes ketones to keep energy levels up. Fasting also works as the early stages of keto when you're not used to it. If you've been eating a high carbohydrate diet, fasting will leave you feeling low on energy and cause brain fog. That's because your body requires time to adjust and make ketones that can be used for energy. If you're already following a ketogenic diet, you aren't going to have near as many problems with this which means that you'll be a lot more comfortable fasting. Your body is already keto-adjusted meaning that you're producing and deriving energy from ketones.

The fact is everyone fasts already! Each day, you go a long time between eating dinner and breakfast. Typically, this period lasts from 8-12 hours or even longer. The word breakfast literally means *breakfast*.

The principles behind intermittent fasting are quite simple. Your body stores excess calories as body fat. It does this because, in the long eons of history that preceded us, people who could call on stored energy to stay alive during periods of food deprivation are the ones who had offspring and passed on their genes. If you couldn't gather energy from stored body fat, you'd be in major trouble if the hunting team couldn't find a deer on a given day.

When you fast, all that happens is your body draws on the reserves of stored fats to produce the energy it needs. Here you can see why those who aren't keto-adapted will find fasting more challenging to deal with. Their bodies aren't used to using ketones to burn energy, and so fasting can make them feel tired, weak, irritable, and bring on brain fog. The bottom line is they get keto flu when they fast.

However, if you've already been doing keto, then your body is already making ketones. It's going to find that using your body fat to get energy is an easy transition.

Having some body fat is normal. A person with zero body fat would be a strange sight indeed, and if they tried fasting, they'd end up burning whatever muscle they had. This is an extreme example but it's one reason that underweight people shouldn't take up fasting. The bottom line is that having some body fat is normal and healthy.

How is body fat created? The body has a natural process that converts excess calories into fat that can be utilized for energy later. It's not all that different than someone who is financially literate and saves for a rainy day.

Let's think about how the financially prepared person conducts their lives. Suppose for simplicity that Sally earns $100 a month.

The person who is careful with their finances realizes that they may not always make $100 a month. They may lose their job, come down with a serious illness, or there may be an economic crisis. They also recognize that in old age if they want to maintain the kind of lifestyle they're used to, they'll need to save money for retirement.

So, Sally plans her life into such a way that she only spends $80 a month on living expenses and entertainment. Each month she puts the excess $20 into her piggy bank. After doing this for three years or 36 months, she has $720 in her piggy bank. This is a stored reserve she can call upon in emergencies, or to use when she retires.

Now consider lazy Joe. He has a job that pays $100 a month too, but he blows all his money. Each month he saves nothing or very little, going out to eat and buying fancy cars. Now and then he puts a few cents in his piggy bank. After three years, he's only got $75 in his bank account.

Then an economic recession hits and both Sally and Joe lose their jobs. Joe is a nervous wreck. He realizes that if he doesn't get a new job fast, he's in big trouble. He starts making plans to sell all his cars, but he can't find buyers because everyone else is hurting too. In a few weeks Joe runs through his $75 and is at the employment office filing for the $10 a month unemployment benefit. Joe, is going to have to curtail his lifestyle in order to survive severely.

Sally, on the other hand, can comfortably spend her money at the same level for several months without worry. She simply looks for a new job and rides out the crisis, living off the funds stored in her piggy bank.

The body is quite similar to this situation. Your body stores fat away when you consume excess calories each day. Of course, unlike finances, some body fat is a good thing but too much causes trouble.

Joe, on the other hand, is like someone who's underweight. They don't have any fat reserves, and so fasting isn't a good deal for them. Joe had to go on unemployment to get *some* money. Like Joe, an underweight person will start burning muscle mass to get some energy. Basically, they will waste away their body.

So how does it actually work?

When you eat food, your body releases insulin along with digestive enzymes. Insulin helps the body take up blood sugar and also acts to help store body fat. There are two major effects:

- Insulin causes sugar to be stored in the liver. It's stored as glycogen and can be released during times of starvation to keep blood sugar levels up. Since glycogen is bound to 3 or 4 water molecules, storing sugar in the liver causes you to put on "water weight."

- Insulin also causes the liver to make fat. The reason is that they livers ability to store glycogen is limited. It can also save some fat, and it can also make fat and then release it into the bloodstream. This latter process is how we get fat.

By now you recognize how everything in the keto puzzle fits together. If you're on keto, you're going to have lower insulin levels, and so your liver will be making less fat.

Remember that the liver has a limited capacity to store glycogen. But we all know that our bodies have an unlimited ability (well virtually unlimited) to store body fat. So, when you're consuming excess calories and your glycogen stores are filled, your body puts the rest away in body fat.

Now that we understand how the body creates and stores fat when excess calories are consumed, let's take a look at what happens when the reverse happens. That is supposed we don't consume any calories at all.

If you're not eating at all, your insulin levels are going to drop. In addition, your blood glucose levels will drop. Your body will then try to find ways to keep your energy levels up, and the first place it's going to look is for glucose. If you're not eating there aren't any outside sources, so your body begins to pull out glycogen, the starches store in your liver (and in muscle cells).

Glycogen can be broken down to make blood sugar and provide energy for the body. Of course, there is a limited supply, so this process only works for a short period. You can exercise too and cut that period way down by burning off all the sugar.

Glycogen stores can power the body for about a day, maybe a day and a half. After that, your body has to call on stored body fat. Most people don't go without food long enough for this process to play out. If you go a few hours without eating, but then replenish your food stores, then you're never going to be in the energy saving mode. At best you'll burn some of the glycogen you have stored.

Intermittent fasting is a way for you to enter the "starvation" state and start burning fat for fuel – your body fat. There are several different methods that people have developed to implement intermittent fasting.

The first method is called 16/8 fasting. This is a pretty simple rule – you limit your eating to 8 hours per day. Then you fast for 16 hours, only consuming water during that time (certainly no alcohol). Since you're eating every day and just restricting the time you consume food to 8 hours, this is a pretty simple way to add fasting to your lifestyle. It's a recommended way for beginners to incorporate fasting.

For example, you can eat dinner between 7:30 PM and 8:00 PM. Then don't eat again until noon the next day. That will give your body a 16 hour fast.

Some experts advise women to use a shorter fasting window, probably 14-15 hours.

The next type of fasting is called 5:2. This is a more advanced and more difficult way to incorporate fasting into your diet. The 5:2 method involves fasting two days per week. It's not necessary to avoid eating at all; practitioners advise consuming a minimal number of calories on fasting days, usually in the range of 500-600 calories.

On the other five days, you eat normally.

So far there hasn't been any scientific proof to demonstrate that 5:2 fasting is better than 16/8 fasting. Moreover, if you're on a ketogenic diet, the benefits of 5:2 fasting are dubious because you're in ketosis already.

The next method of fasting is popularly known as *eat, stop eat.* This involves a complete 24 hour fast. You can choose when to start your 24-hour fast, but it's recommended that you start after eating dinner one night and then don't eat again for 24 hours. You can do this once or twice a week.

This fits in with keto better than the 5:2 method and seems to be quite effective, but may be too much for a lot of people. During the 24-hour fasting period, you don't consume any food products. Simply drink water. For many people, this type of fasting will require a great deal of discipline.

Alternate day fasting involves fasting one day and then eating the next. Some practitioners of this type of fasting follow the 5:2 plan of eating about 500 calories on fasting days. Of course, if you're consuming food, you're not really fasting.

The *warrior diet* is a variation of the 24-hour fasting plan. Using the warrior diet, you only eat once per day. You're advised to consume a large meal, so that you get all of your calories in one sitting. You probably don't want to do this at breakfast, but can do it at lunch or dinner. It's generally advised that you eat your big meal at dinner so that you're consuming all of your calories before going to sleep for the night, so will save some for the next day. The idea is to put your body in a fasting state so that the excess is burned off during the daytime when you're not eating.

There are many different methods of intermittent fasting, and you might have to experiment to see what works best in your case since we're all different. However, it's important to note that with keto the extreme methods of fasting aren't generally necessary. When you're on keto, you're already burning ketones, and have also already depleted excess glycogen stores.

Possible Benefits from Fasting

Let's begin with the obvious. If you engage in intermittent fasting, you're consuming fewer calories. So, you'll experience some level of weight loss. You can accelerate your keto diet plan by adding some intermittent fasting.

It's long been believed that fasting was a way to 'detoxify' the body. That perception is largely correct. Even if you're not eliminating specific 'toxins,' fasting helps detoxify the body in subtle but important ways.

One of the most important ways is that it helps you maintain lower and more stable blood sugar levels. Your insulin level is also reduced. So, in a sense, you're detoxifying your body from its toxins. Insulin isn't really a toxin, but too much of it has toxic effects on the body.

If done properly, intermittent fasting will help you specifically lost body fat. You shouldn't go right into intermittent fasting if you're a keto beginner, as you can lower your glycogen stores simply by adopting a keto diet. Then you'll be able to use intermittent fasting to accelerate the loss of excess body fat.

If you want to do one of the more extreme fasting methods, you can gradually ease into it. Consider starting with the 16/8 method. This is something that most people will be pretty comfortable doing, especially after they're in ketosis. Then one day per week, you can gradually expand the time fasting. The first time you might go 17/7, and then work up to 16/6. The goal is to reach a full 24 hour fast once per week eventually. After you've done that you can add a second day of 24-hour fasting if desired.

While you need to check with your doctor first, doing intermittent fasting can have dramatic effects on those who have type 2 diabetes. Fasting can have major impacts that stabilize blood sugar levels and reduce your blood sugar. Some people even claim to cure their diabetes using intermittent fasting in combination with a ketogenic diet.

Some other benefits that people have associated with intermittent fasting include:

- Weight loss
- Lower blood sugar and cholesterol
- Lower insulin levels
- Burning fat and not muscle
- Increased mental clarity (probably comes from utilizing ketones)
- Increased growth hormones
- Reduced triglycerides

Another possible benefit is the so-called Autophagy. This is a cellular process that involves what might be described as a home cleaning. Your body's immune machinery will go through the body and clear out all the old dysfunctional cells. It is believed that intermittent fasting may trigger or increase this process, helping you achieve a healthier state.

Determining If Fasting Is for You

It's important to note that fasting is not for everyone. It takes discipline and at first, it's going to make you feel tired, irritable and uncomfortable. We will note however that if you're already doing the keto diet, the negative consequences of fasting will be minimized if you experience them at all.

First, let's review who should not be fasting. Frankly, the list of people who should not be fasting include:

- Type 1 diabetics
- Type 2 diabetics on insulin or drugs like metformin that manage blood sugar levels
- Underweight people
- People with serious illnesses like cancer

Well, we've been a little to absolutist. It's possible for type 2 diabetics to engage in fasting, but you should talk about it with your doctor first and adjust your medications and dosing schedule as necessary. The same advice applies to those with cancer, although recent research has rediscovered the fact that cancer cells feed on sugar, so depriving your cancer cells might assist in your treatment plan. Again, talk to your doctor if this describes your situation.

Beyond a few specific subgroups of people, determining if fasting for you is a matter of taste. It's important to note that you don't need to fast to get results from a ketogenic diet, but fasting may speed the results you're looking for and help you maintain a healthier lifestyle.

If you're unsure about fasting but are interested in it, the best thing to do is try to work it in gradually and see how your body reacts. As noted in the previous section, you can slowly ease your way into a 24 hour fast. Alternatively, simply to 16/8 fasting. This method of fasting –when done in conjunction with a keto diet – is pretty gentle. If you do not have diabetes on insulin, you can do 16/8 fasting without giving it any thought. You probably won't even know you're fasting once you've been on the keto diet for any length of time.

Thinking about ketosis, you can see why 16/8 fasting would give a person eating a "normal" diet the blues. When you're eating a diet with a large amount of carbohydrates and not on ketosis, you need to feed yourself sugar to keep going continually. People eating carbs get hungry and they have to eat more often. If you're doing keto one of the first things you might notice is that you're not having hunger pains anymore.

But if you're still eating "normally," your body continually experiences blood sugar peaks and crashes. Through the night your blood sugar gradually drops (unless your pre-diabetic or diabetic, but remember they have trouble using their blood sugar for energy). So, in the morning people are often famished and need to eat and get their blood sugar back up. Far too many people make things even worse by consuming sweets with breakfast, eating sugar-laden donuts or breakfast cereals. And remember even so-called "whole grains" are nothing but sugar, it's just packaged in such a way that it's a little bit harder to get to so takes longer to digest. Whole grains might result in blood sugar spikes that come on more gradually and last longer – but they still create a rise in blood sugar. That simple fact can't be avoided.

Keep in mind that fasting means fasting. You don't want to ruin it by consuming any calories. If you find you need to drink coffee while fasting, you'll have to do it without cream and sweetener (and never sugar –fasting or not). It's best to stick to water while fasting.

If getting up in the morning and going without your coffee and cream is too much to bear, consider doing a 16/8 plan where your 8 hours of eating begins at 8 or 9 in the morning. Just remember that you'll have to schedule your last meal accordingly. If you start consuming at 9 AM, you'll have to be done eating by 5 PM.

Many will find that an occasional 24 hour fast works better for them. You can limit this to one day per week if you find that the impact is too stressful. In any case, plan ahead and test and retest.

- First, get yourself adjusted to keto. Don't start fasting until you're in ketosis and have gotten over the "keto flu" if it's impacting you.

- Try the 16/8 fasting plan first. It's very easy to implement. But remember if you wait until noon to eat your first meal but have morning coffee with cream, you're not fasting. Fasting means not consuming any calories.

- Experiment with different methods. Some people will benefit from or tolerate different ways of fasting.

- The advantage of a once or twice a week fast, or a 5:2 style of fasting, is that you're not fasting all the time.

- If fasting isn't really your thing, but you'd like to enjoy the benefits, try occasionally fasting. Maybe you only fast for 24 hours once or twice a month. It's not necessary to fast all the time to get the benefits.

Chapter 13: The Keto Breakfast

Keto means a lot of cooking. But my meal plan and shopping list will make this the most fun part of the diet. Cooking healthy meals that taste good and are wholly satisfying not only feeds the body, it feeds the soul. Treat yourself and sit down to well-prepared keto meals made with the highest quality ingredients you can afford. It makes a difference, I assure you.

What follows is a 7-day plan. Your first week of keto dieting already planned so you can effortlessly transition without the stress of thinking of *what to cook next*. I have even included a list that will take the guesswork out of grocery shopping. Use the weekend to prep as many ingredients as possible. Wash, chop and store vegetables. Cook and divide meat into servings ready to go. Boil all the eggs at once. Gather spill-proof containers to bring all your keto yumminess to the workplace.

Once you get the hang of cooking and eating keto, you'll be able to mix the recipes around and add a few of your own. The key to healthy eating is variety, which is as we all know, is the spice of life.

In this chapter, we'll cover a seven-day breakfast plan with recipes.

Monday
Breakfast: Simple scrambled eggs with tomato slices

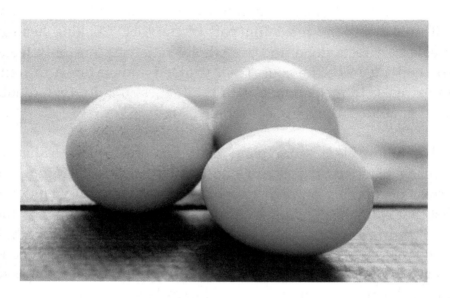

This recipe combines high-quality protein with a low carb tomato to keep you fuller longer.

Variation tip: Substitute your favorite low carb vegetable like spinach or avocado.

Prep Time: 5 minutes
Cook Time: 5 minutes
Servings: 1

What's in it
- Butter (1 ounce)
- Eggs (2)
- Water (1 T)
- Salt and pepper (to taste)
- Small whole tomato (1 qty)

How it's made

- Heat the butter over medium heat in a 10-inch non-stick skillet.
- Crack the eggs into a bowl, add water and beat lightly with a whisk.
- Add the eggs to the skillet and stir until just firm. Be careful not to overcook.
- Slice tomato and serve with the eggs.
- Season with salt and pepper.

Net carbs: 5 grams
Fat: 15 grams
Protein: 11 grams
Sugars: 2.6 grams

Tuesday
Breakfast: Avocado salmon boats

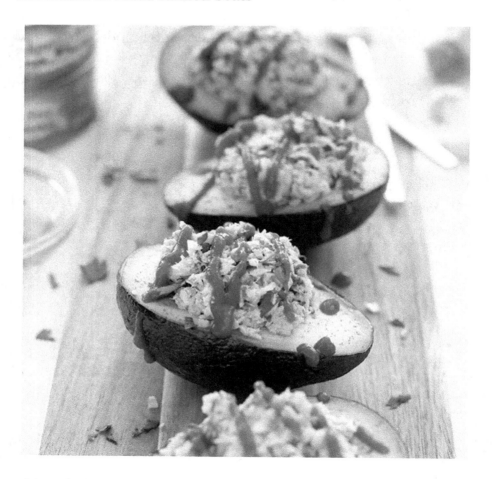

This wholesome breakfast requires no cooking at all, but it's delicious and packed with protein and good fats.

Variation tip: try sour cream instead of mayo.

Prep Time: 5 minutes
Cook Time: None
Servings: 2

What's in it
- Avocados (2 qty)
- Wild caught smoked salmon (6 ounces)
- Mayonnaise (4 T)
- Salt and pepper (to taste)
- Lemon (1 qty)

How it's made
- Carefully cut avocadoes in half. Remove pits.
- Add a tablespoon of sour cream or mayonnaise in the hollow of each avocado half.
- Top each half with equal amounts of salmon
- Sprinkle with salt and pepper
- Cut the lemon into quarters and squeeze over each boat before serving.

Net carbs: 1 gram
Fat: 71 grams
Protein: 16 grams
Sugars: 1 gram

Wednesday
Breakfast: Simple Egg Salad

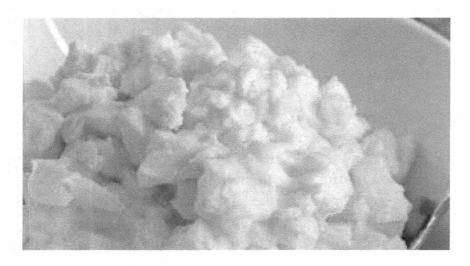

Egg butter is a savory, flavorful way to start your day.

Variation tip: mix in a little fresh dill or chives.

Prep Time: 5 minutes
Cook Time: 10 minutes
Serves 2

What's in it

- Eggs (4 qty)
- Butter (5 ounces)
- Kosher salt (.5 tsp.)
- Fresh ground pepper (.25 t)

How it's made

- Place eggs in a large pot and fill to cover with cold, filtered water.

- Bring to a rolling boil and let cook for 8-minutes.
- Carefully drain eggs and plunge into a bowl of ice water to stop the eggs from overcooking.
- After the eggs have cooled, peel and chop.
- Combine with butter, kosher salt and fresh ground pepper
- Goes great with lettuce leaves. Also try with avocado slices, smoked salmon, turkey, or ham.

Net carbs: 1 gram
Fat: 69 grams
Protein: 12 grams
Sugars: None

Thursday
Breakfast: Pancakes, The Keto Way

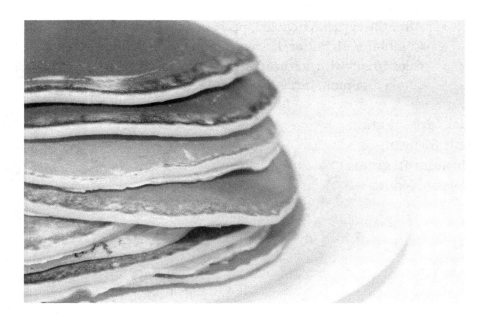

What a treat! Pancakes on the keto diet. If you thought you would miss fluffy pancakes, then try these. They're delicious.

Variation tip: serve with berries and homemade whipped cream, peanut butter or even crumpled, crispy bacon.

Prep Time: 5 minutes
Cook Time: 10 minutes
Serves 4

What's in it
- Eggs (4 qty)
- Cottage cheese (7 ounces)
- Ground psyllium husk powder (At healthy grocery stores 1T)
- Butter (2 ounces)

How it's made

- Mix eggs, cheese and psyllium husk powder together and set aside. The mixture will thicken.
- Over medium heat, melt butter in a nonstick skillet. When melted and slightly bubbly, pour 3 T of pancake batter and cook for 4 minutes. Flip and cook for 3 more minutes. Proceed with the rest of the batter.

Net carbs: 5 grams
Fat: 39 grams
Protein: 13 grams
Sugars: 2 grams

Friday
Breakfast: Break the Fast Burrito Bowl

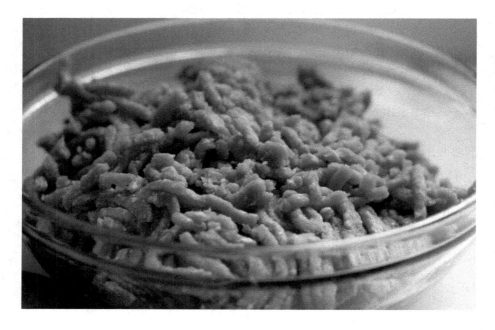

Skip the carbs from the tortilla by putting leftover seasoned beef and veggies into a bowl. So easy.

Variation tip: try different toppings, like salsa.

Prep Time: 5 minutes
Cook Time: 15 minutes
Serves 2

What's in it
- Seasoned ground beef – can use Keto Taco recipe (.5 pounds)
- Prepared riced cauliflower (2 cups)
- Chopped cilantro (2 T)
- Butter (2 t, divided)

- Eggs (3 qty)
- Salt (to taste)
- Pepper (to taste)

How it's made
- Brown and season the beef in a large skillet with a teaspoon of the butter. When done, push to one side.
- Add diced cauliflower and chopped cilantro. Season with salt. Push to the side.
- Melt a teaspoon of butter in the open space of the skillet.
- Beat the eggs and add to the butter. Scramble in the skillet. If your skillet isn't large enough for this step, use a separate pan.
- Mix everything together. Taste.
- Season with salt and pepper if necessary.

Net carbs: 4 grams
Fat: 14 grams
Protein: 34 grams
Sugars: 2 grams

Saturday
Breakfast: Jalapeno Bacon Egg Cups

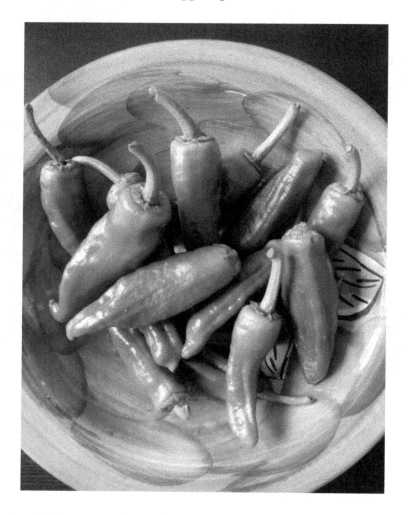

Have a little extra time this morning for some self-care? Try my Jalapeno Bacon Egg Cups. These spicy cups will wake your senses and send you out the door with a spring in your step.

Variation tip: replace jalapenos with green onions.

Prep Time: 5 minutes
Cook Time: 20 minutes
Serves 4

What's in it
- Nitrate-free bacon, cooked and crumbled (5 ounces)
- Eggs (12 qty)
- Cheddar, shredded (6 ounces)
- Jalapeno (2 qty)
- Salt (to taste)
- Pepper (to taste)

How it's made
- Turn the oven on so that it preheats to 350 degrees F.
- Cut jalapeno in half, lengthwise, and remove seeds. Chop 1 jalapeno and slice the other.
- Beat eggs with a whisk and add cheese
- Grease a muffin tin with fat of choice and layer the bottom with the chopped jalapeno and bacon. Pour the egg mixture into each muffin well.
- Each muffin gets a slice of the other jalapeno on top.
- Pop into the hot oven for about 20 minutes. Eggs should no longer look wet. When done, remove from oven and let cool.
- Serve

Net carbs: 3 grams
Fat: 39 grams
Protein: 35 grams
Sugars: 0 grams

Sunday
Breakfast: Classic bacon and eggs for one

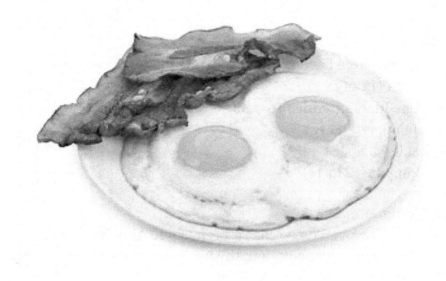

What's it in it (for one):
- 2 eggs
- 1¼ oz. bacon, in slices
- cherry tomatoes (optional)
- fresh parsley (optional)

How it's made:
- Fry bacon in a pan on medium-high heat. Remove and set aside, leaving bacon fat in the pan.
- Crack eggs and place in pan, cooking and seasoning to taste. You can cook them scrambled, sunny side up or any way you like. Optionally you can add a small bit of cream to up the fat content of your meal and add extra flavor.
- Slice cherry tomatoes in half, and optionally quickly fry in the bacon grease.

- Put the entire contents of the pan onto your serving plate. Optionally, substitute two strawberries or blackberries for the cherry tomatoes.

Net carbs: 1 gram
Fat: 22 grams
Protein: 15 grams
Sugars: 0 grams but depends on optional fruits or vegetables

Chapter 14: The Keto Lunch

In this chapter, we'll provide a seven-day menu that you can use for some easy to make but extremely delicious keto lunches.

Monday
Lunch: Keto Meatballs

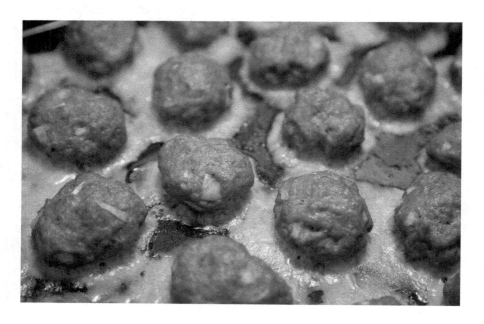

Make these ahead of time because these delicious meatballs are freezable. Take a few to work along with some sugar-free marinara sauce and zoodles (zucchini noodles) for a delicious keto lunch.

Variation tip: change the seasonings to make different flavors, like taco or barbecue.

Prep Time: 5 minutes
Cook Time: 18 minutes
Servings: 4

What's in it

- Grass-fed ground beef (1 pound)
- Chopped fresh parsley (1.5 t)
- Onion powder (.75 t)
- Garlic powder (.75 t)
- Kosher salt (.75 t)
- Fresh ground black pepper (.5 t)

How it's made

- Turn oven to 400-degrees F to preheat.
- Using parchment paper, line a baking sheet.
- Put beef into a medium-sized glass bowl with other ingredients and mix with hands until just combined. Avoid over-mixing as this will result in tough meatballs.
- Roll into 8 meatballs and place on the lined baking sheet.
- Bake for 15-18 minutes until done all the way through.

Net carbs: 3 grams
Fat: 17 grams
Protein: 11 grams
Sugars: 2 grams

Tuesday
Lunch: Mason Jar Salad

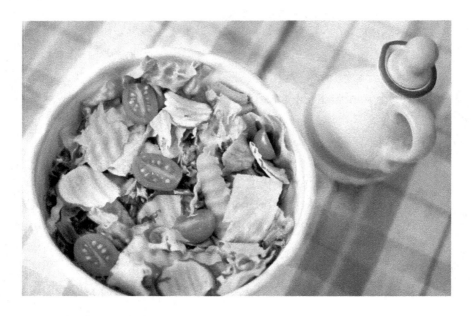

So colorful and full of flavor. This salad is portable. Use any vegetable you have on hand.

Variation tip: try different kinds of protein, cheese or seeds.

Prep Time: 10 minutes
Cook Time: None
Servings: 1

What's in it
- Cooked, diced chicken (4 ounces)
- Baby spinach (1/6 ounce)
- Cherry tomatoes (1/6 ounce)
- Bell pepper (1/6 ounce)
- Cucumber (1/6 ounce)
- Green onion (1/2 qty)

- Extra virgin olive oil (4 T)

How it's made
- Chop vegetables.
- Stuff spinach at the bottom of jar.
- Layer the rest of the vegetables.
- Keep olive oil in a separate container until ready to eat.

Net carbs: 4 grams
Fat: 55 grams
Protein: 71 grams
Sugars: 1 gram

Wednesday

Lunch: The Smoked Salmon Special

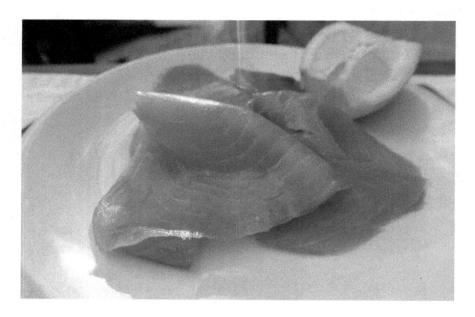

This may be the easiest lunch special ever. Flavorful, smoky, pink salmon poses on your plate next to dark, green spinach as a feast for the eyes and the body.

Variation tip: serve with arugula or cabbage.

Prep Time: 5 minutes
Cook Time: None
Serves 2

What's in it
- Wild caught smoked salmon (.5 ounces)
- Mayonnaise (generous dollop)
- Baby spinach (large handful)
- Extra virgin olive oil (.5 T)
- Lime wedge (1 qty)

- Kosher salt (to taste)
- Fresh ground pepper (to taste)

How it's made
- Place salmon (or any fatty fish like sardines or mackerel) and spinach on a plate.
- Add a large spoonful of mayonnaise and the lime wedge.
- Drizzle oil atop the baby spinach (or try arugula or cabbage shredded as if for slaw)
- Sprinkle with a little salt and pepper.

Net carbs: None
Fat: 109 grams
Protein: 105 grams
Sugars: None

Thursday
Lunch: Ham and Brie Plate

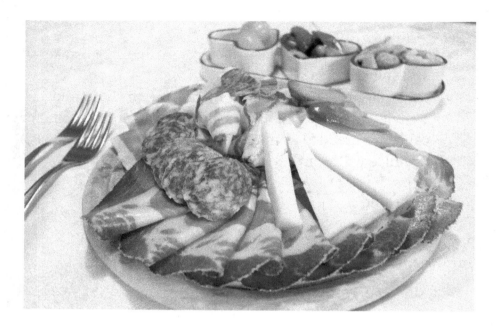

Like a hoagie, but way better.

Variation tip: this is a mix-and-match situation, so experiment with different cheeses and cold cuts.

Prep Time: 5 minutes
Cook Time: None
Serves 2

What's in it
- Ham, sliced thin (9 ounces)
- Brie cheese (5 ounces)
- Anchovies (2/3 ounces
- Green pesto (2 T)
- Kalamata olives (10 qty)

- Baby spinach (1/6 ounce)
- Mayonnaise (.5 cup)
- Fresh basil leaves (10 qty)

How it's made
- Place ingredients on a plate with a serving of mayonnaise.

Net carbs: 6 grams
Fat: 103 grams
Protein: 40 grams
Sugars: 0 grams

Friday
Lunch: Creamy Avocado and Bacon with Goat Cheese Salad

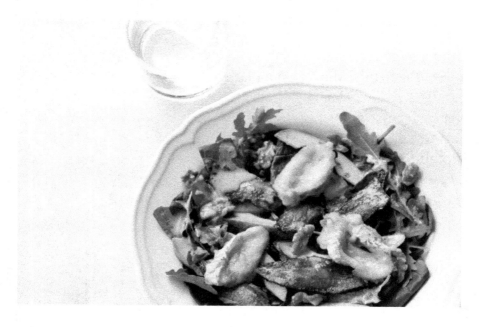

Salad gets an upgrade when crave-able avocado and goat cheese are combined with crispy bacon and crunchy nuts. Fast and good for lunch or dinner.

Variation tip: use different fresh herbs in the dressing.

Prep Time: 10 minutes
Cook Time: 20 minutes
Serves 4

What's in it
Salad:

- Goat cheese (1 8-ounce log)
- Bacon (.5 pound)
- Avocados (2 qty)
- Toasted walnuts or pecans (.5 cup)

- Arugula or baby spinach (4 ounces)

Dressing:
- One-half lemon, juiced
- Mayonnaise (.5 cup)
- Extra virgin olive oil (.5 cup)
- Heavy whipping cream (2 T)
- Kosher salt (to taste)
- Fresh ground pepper (to taste)

How it's made
- Line a baking dish with parchment paper.
- Preheat oven to 400 degrees F.
- Slice goat cheese into half-inch rounds and put in baking dish. Place on an upper rack in preheated oven until golden brown.
- Cook bacon until crisp. Chop into pieces
- Slice avocado and place on greens. Top with bacon pieces and add goat cheese rounds.
- Chop nuts and sprinkle on the salad.
- For dressing, combine lemon juice, mayo, extra virgin olive oil and whipping cream. Blend with countertop or immersion blender.
- Season to taste with kosher salt and fresh ground pepper.

Net carbs: 6 grams
Fat: 123 grams
Protein: 27 grams
Sugars: 1 gram

Saturday
Lunch: Chicken Noodle-less Soup

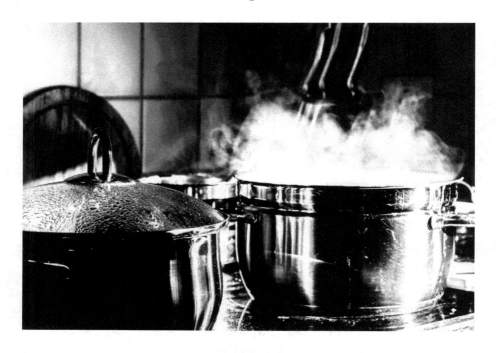

All the comfort of a classic soup without the carbs. How comforting.

Variation tip: use the meat from a rotisserie chicken.

Prep Time: 10 minutes
Cook Time: 20 minutes
Serves 4

What's in it
- Butter (.25 cup)
- Celery (1 stalk)
- Mushrooms (3 ounces)
- Garlic, minced (1 clove)

- Dried minced onion (1 T)
- Dried parsley (1 t)
- Chicken stock (4 cups)
- Kosher salt (.5 t)
- Fresh ground pepper (.25 t)
- Carrot, chopped (1 qty)
- Chicken, cooked and diced (2.5 cups or 1.5 pounds of chicken breast)
- Cabbage, sliced (1 cups)

How it's made
- Put large soup pot on medium heat and melt butter.
- Slice the celery and mushrooms and add, along with dried onion to the pot.
- Add parsley, broth, carrot, kosher salt and fresh pepper. Stir.
- Simmer until veggies are tender.
- Stir in cooked chicken and sliced cabbage. Simmer until cabbage is tender, about 8 to 12 minutes.

Net carbs: 4 grams
Fat: 40 grams
Protein: 33 grams
Sugars: 1 gram

Sunday
Lunch: Cheese and turkey rollups

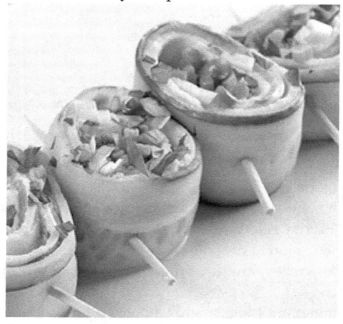

What's in it:
- 3 slices of turkey lunchmeat
- 3 slices of cheese (your choice)
- ½ avocado
- 3 slices of cucumber
- a quarter cup of blueberries
- handful of almonds

How it's made:

- Using your cheese as bread, make "turkey rolls" by rolling up the turkey meat, a few slices of avocado, and the cucumber slices.
- Enjoy, and snack on the blueberries and almonds.

Contains 13 net carbs.

Chapter 15: Keto at Dinner

Monday

Dinner: Beef short ribs in a slow cooker

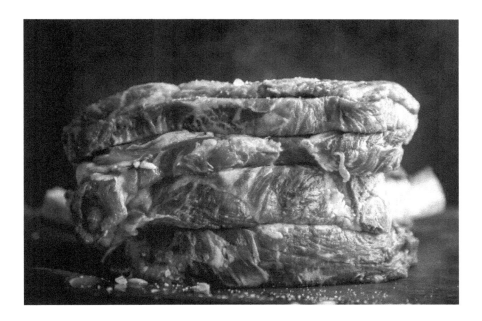

With a little prep, you will have a hot meal waiting for you at the end of a long day.

Variation tip: serve over diced cauliflower or with celery.

Prep Time: 15 minutes
Cook Time: 4 hours
Servings: 4

What's in it
- Boneless short ribs or bone-in (2 pounds)
- Kosher salt (to taste)
- Fresh ground pepper (to taste)

- Extra virgin olive oil (2 T)
- Chopped white onion (1 qty)
- Garlic (3 cloves)
- Bone broth (1 cup)
- Coconut aminos (2 T)
- Tomato paste (2 T)
- Red wine (1.5 cups)

How it's made
- In a large skillet over medium heat, add olive oil. Season meat with salt and pepper. Brown both sides.
- Add broth and browned ribs to slow cooker
- Put remaining ingredients into the skillet.
- Bring to a boil and cook until onions are tender. About 5 minutes.
- Pour over ribs.
- Set to 4 to 6 hours on high or 8 to 10 hours on low.

Net carbs: 1 gram
Fat: 63 grams
Protein: 24 grams
Sugars: 1 gram

Tuesday
Dinner: Chicken Thighs with Garlic and Parmesan Cheese

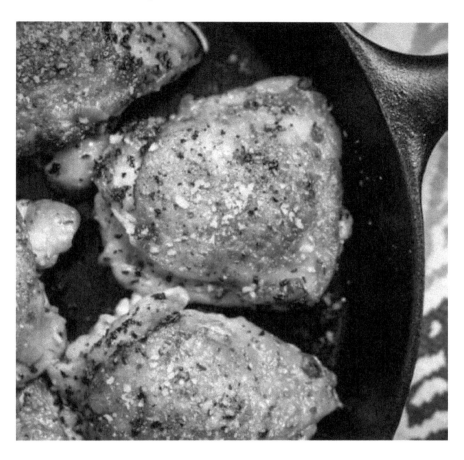

Tastes like chicken wings but heartier.

Variation tip: try cooking in a cast iron skillet for superb searing. Dried basil instead of Italian seasoning would work nicely.

Prep Time: 5 minutes
Cook Time: 35 minutes
Serves 4

What's in it
- Bone in chicken thighs (6 qty)
- Italian seasoning (1 T)
- Shredded parmesan cheese (1 T)
- Garlic cloves, chopped (1 qty)
- Kosher salt (to taste)
- Fresh ground pepper (to taste)

How it's made
- Turn oven to 450 degrees F to preheat
- Pull the skin away from the top of the thigh to create a pocket.
- Mix together Italian seasoning, shredded parmesan cheese, garlic, 1/8 teaspoon of kosher salt, fresh ground pepper and scant drops of extra virgin olive oil.
- Divide the mixture between the thighs. Rub evenly under the skin.
- In an ovenproof skillet, heat extra virgin olive oil over medium-high heat.
- Put thighs skin side down and allow to cook for about 5 minutes. Flip and cook for 8 to 10 minutes.
- Transfer the skillet to the hot oven for 15-20 minutes until cooked all the way through.
- Let rest, then serve.

Net carbs: 0.6 grams
Fat: 29 grams
Protein: 27 grams
Sugars: 0 grams

Wednesday
Dinner: Keto Tacos

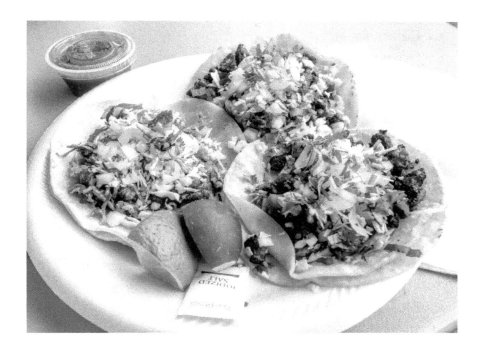

Tacos get a makeover too. Instead of tortillas, filling is stuffed into zucchini boats. Make extra seasoning to always have on hand for taco meat anytime.

Variation tips: Try different types of cheeses. Serve with salsa.

Prep Time: 15 minutes
Cook Time: 30 minutes
Serves 4

What's in it
- Zucchini (2 qty)
- Extra virgin olive oil (3 T, divided)
- Grass fed ground beef or pork (1 pound)

- Kosher salt (1 t)
- White onion, chopped (.25 cup)
- Chili powder (1 t)
- Cumin (.5 t)
- Oregano (.5 t)
- Shredded cheddar cheese (1.25 cups)

How it's made
- Turn oven to 400 degrees F to preheat.
- Slice zucchini in half lengthwise and scoop out seeds to make boats. Sprinkle with kosher salt. Let sit for about 10 minutes.
- Heat 2 T of extra virgin olive oil in skillet and brown meat.
- Add chili powder, cumin, oregano and salt. Cook until liquid is mostly gone.
- Blot zucchini with a paper towel and put on a baking sheet that has been greased.
- Mix 1/3 of cheese in the seasoned beef.
- Stuff the cheesy beef into the zucchini boats evenly and place in hot oven for about 20 minutes until cheese starts to turn brown. Remove from the oven and let cool for a few minutes.

Net carbs: 6 grams
Fat: 49 grams
Protein: 33 grams
Sugars: 2 grams

Thursday

Dinner: On the go chicken wings with green beans

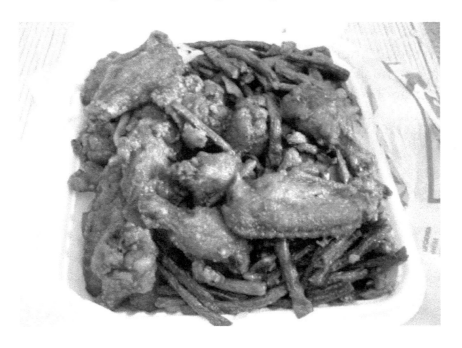

We decided to incorporate a meal idea here to illustrate how you can build your keto meals when you're pressed for time.

What's In it:
- Pecan smoked chicken wings (frozen, available at WalMart)
- Marketside French Green beans (fresh and packaged for microwaving, available at Walmart.

How it's made:
- Preheat oven to 425.
- Bake chicken wings for 30-35 minutes.
- When chicken wings are almost done, place beans inside a microwave in the bag and cook for 2-3 minutes.

- Take beans out and season with butter or olive oil, and salt and pepper.
- Enjoy with your chicken wings!

Net carbs: 7 grams
Fat: 14 grams per 4 ounces serving of chicken, be sure to add butter or olive oil used
Protein: 14 grams per 4 ounces serving of chicken
Sugars: 3 grams

Friday
Dinner: Minute Steak with Mushrooms and Herb Butter

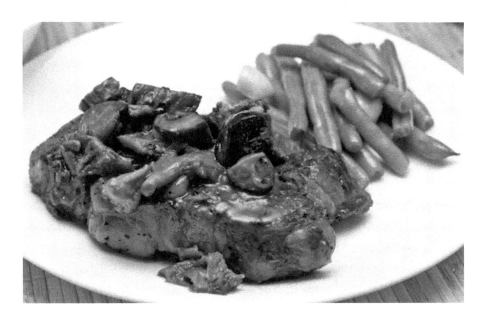

This dinner comes together fast. Perfect for busy weeknights.

Variation tip: try over any of your favorite vegetables.

Prep Time: 10 minutes
Cook Time: 20 minutes
Serves 4

What's in it
For steaks:
- Minute steaks (8 qty)
- Toothpicks (8 qty)
- Gruyere cheese, cut into sticks (3 ounces)
- Kosher salt (to taste)
- Fresh ground pepper (to taste)
- Butter (2 T)

- Leeks (2 qty)
- Mushrooms (15 ounces)
- Extra virgin olive oil (2 T)

For herb butter:

- Butter (5 ounces)
- Minced garlic cloves (1 qty)
- Garlic powder (.5 T)
- Chopped parsley (4 T)
- Lemon juice (1 t)
- Kosher salt (.5 t)

How it's made

- Combine all herb butter ingredients in a glass bowl. Set aside for at least 15 minutes.
- Slice leeks and mushrooms. Sauté in extra virgin olive oil until lightly brown. Season with salt and pepper. Remove from skillet and keep warm.
- Season steaks with salt and pepper. Place a stick of cheese in the center and roll up steaks, securing with a toothpick.
- Sauté on medium heat for 10 to 15 minutes.
- Pour pan juices on vegetables.
- Plate steaks and vegetables and serve with herb butter.

Net carbs: 6 grams
Fat: 89 grams
Protein: 52 grams
Sugars: 2 grams

Saturday
Dinner: "Breaded" Pork Chops

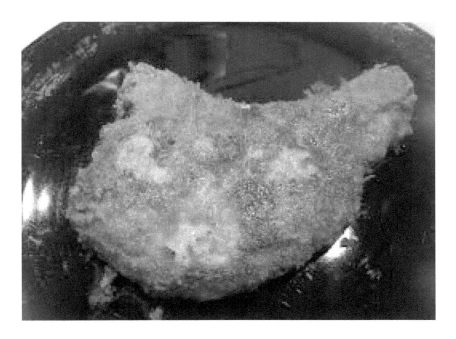

With crispy, keto friendly breading, this is sure to be a family favorite.

Variation tip: if you can spare the calories, sprinkle with shredded Parmesan cheese.

Prep Time: 5 minutes
Cook Time: 30 minutes
Serves 4

What's in it

- Boneless thin pork chops (4 qty)
- Psyllium husk powder (1 T)
- Kosher salt (.5 t)
- Paprika (.25 t)

- Garlic powder (.25 t)
- Onion powder (.25 t)
- Oregano (.25 t)

How it's made

- Preheat oven to 350 degrees F.
- Dry pork chops with a paper towel.
- Combine the rest of the ingredients in a ziplock bag.
- One at a time, seal the pork chops in the bag and shake to coat.
- Put a wire rack on a baking sheet. Place pork chops on rack.
- Bake in oven for approximately 30 minutes. The thermometer should read 145 degrees F.
- Serve with vegetables or a green salad.

Net carbs: 0 grams
Fat: 9 grams
Protein: 28 grams
Sugars: 0 grams

Sunday
Dinner: Lamb Chops

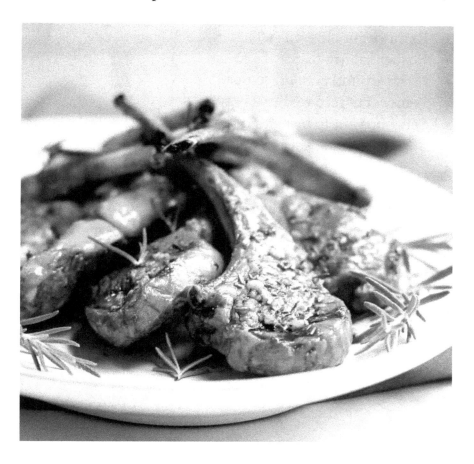

Celebrate Saturday night with juicy lamb chops served with herbal butter. Perfection.

Variation tip: serve with a simple green salad or other vegetable. Can also substitute pork chops.

Prep Time: 15 minutes
Cook Time: 10 minutes
Serves 4

What's in it
- Lamb chops (8 qty)
- Butter (1 T)
- Extra virgin olive oil (1 T)
- Kosher salt (to taste)
- Fresh ground pepper (to taste)
- Lemon, cut into wedges (1 qty)
- Set chops out to bring to room temperature.
- Sprinkle with kosher salt and fresh ground pepper.
- Heat butter and oil in skillet. Add chops and brown on both sides, 3 to 4 minutes each side.
- Serve with lemon wedges and butter.

Net carbs: 1 gram
Fat: 90 grams
Protein: 44 grams
Sugars: 0 gram

Chapter 16: Eating on the Go

One of the pitfalls facing beginners on the keto diet is eating with other people – this can include eating at home with family members who don't want to join you on keto or going out to eat. We leave it to the reader to work out how they're going to deal with their family members – in this chapter we'll offer some remarks and guidance about eating out.

Managing Keto in Restaurants

There are many distinct issues that you'll be dealing with while eating out. Many of them are so obvious they're not even worth discussing, but for the sake of completeness, we'll mention them. Obviously, you're going to want to avoid eating carbohydrate laden meals. That means to hold the French fries. A medium serving of McDonalds French fries contains 50 grams of carbs. So, eat that and you're done – you've gone way beyond any permissible limits on carbohydrate consumption when it comes to keto. Only 4.6 grams of a medium order of French fries are dietary fiber – so they pack on with net carbs too.

Luckily for us, we not only live in a time when food is convenient and widely available, but we also live in an era when information is king. This will be harder with local restaurants, but large ones and chains have posted complete nutritional information online. Use this information. You can build up a nice detailed list of where you can eat and what you can eat, and how much damage eating a particular place will do to your diet.

Unfortunately, there are not many restaurants that cater to keto, paleo, or low carb eating. So, you're going to have to adapt to them rather than the other way around. One option you can consider if one is located near your office or home is Boston

Market. You'll have to be careful on the side items – but Boston Market offers quarter and half chickens and other meat items like prime rib.

Barbecue places can also be utilized (but more below). You can consume a lot of meat items like chicken, pork ribs, and beef brisket.

One surprising option that might surprise you is fried chicken. Now we offer this with a caveat – we are not suggesting that you should include fried chicken with your keto diet. But if you're in a bind and need some fast food, it might be an option.

For example, according to the Church's Chicken website, they list the following carbohydrate content:

- Leg: 6 carbs
- Wing: 8 carbs
- Thigh: 12 carbs (1 gram of fiber, 11 net carbs)
- Breast: 9 carbs

So, it's possible to eat a meal of fried chicken without completely wrecking your diet. Of course, having more than one piece comes dangerously close – you'll have to watch your vegetable consumption the rest of the day to stay under 30 grams of total carbs.

In hamburger joints, you can always eat the burger without the bun. You can also opt for steak or fish in many restaurants, and only eat vegetables. In Mexican restaurants, if they have it available eat carne asada or carne adovada, which is beef or pork in a spicy sauce that usually has little or no carbohydrates.

In an Indian restaurant, you can opt for kabobs. Note that depending on the local recipe used tandoori chicken might have a lot of carbohydrates. Food items like Chinese are usually entirely out. If you want to eat Chinese, you'll have to consider it on a cheat day.

Sushi can work and can be a healthy option for keto dieters. If you're going to do sushi though you'll need to restrict yourself to *sashimi*, which is plain raw fish. Soy sauce and wasabi are OK to use. Stay away from soups and "salads" that might be enhanced with carbohydrates or sweetened with sugar.

The bottom line is that eating out is very difficult on keto, as the rest of the world hasn't come around to this healthy lifestyle, at least not yet. So, it's probably best to pack a lunch for work or school. If you have to eat out, you might use a keto meter to track directly and see how your body is responding, and what meals cause you to go off ketosis and which ones don't. By process of trial and error you might find some meals that work for you.

Watch Out for Hidden Carbs

If you do find yourself in a position where you have to eat out, one of the biggest dangers is hidden carbs. While everyone else is worrying about butter, they aren't noticing that the chefs are using sugar and starches to "spice up" their food.

Some of these hidden carbs are more obvious than others. The first place where you're going to find hidden carbs is in condiments and sauces. Barbecue sauce as many people know is loaded with sugar. On a teaspoon by teaspoon basis, you're not getting a huge amount of sugar, but if you eat food marinated in different sauces, there is no telling how much you're consuming. On keto, it's important to know how many carbs you're getting.

Another problem is the teriyaki sauce. You can hit a Japanese restaurant and say "hold the rice" but teriyaki sauce has sugar in it, and the amount of sugar will vary. If it's a larger restaurant or chain, you may be able to find out how much sugar is in the sauce, but in most cases it's a guessing game.

Pizza, of course, is completely out. And it's not just the tomato sauce.

Chines food, like Japanese, can be problematic. You might be able to find some dishes that without the rice appear to be meat and vegetables. Two problems come up here – the first is that you're not getting enough fat. What do most Chinese dishes include? Lean meat. Of course, there are oils in the sauces but the second issue is that Chinese sauces usually contain a lot of sugar.

In fact, cooked vegetables in any restaurant can be a problem. Remember restaurants don't care about your health, they only care about creating addicting food that tastes good. So, the "vegetables" might be cooked in a sugar-containing sauce or marinade and it might not be immediately evident that this was done. So, you might be consuming more carbs than you think you are.

Not to be brutal about it, but the bottom line is no matter what eating out can be problematic. It might not be feasible to avoid eating out all the time, but a good rule for a beginner to follow is to use the plan put forward by the Atkins diet. Take at least two weeks (the "induction" phase) where your carbohydrates are severely restricted to twenty grams per day. You can do this for two weeks or up to a month depending on your situation. After that, then you can ease up a bit and start eating out now and then. That way you'll achieve your weight loss goals and not suffer a catastrophic defeat by eating out once in a while.

We've also discussed the possibility of incorporating a "cheat" day here and there. This should also be done after the induction period, but if you include a cheat day, you can schedule it, so it occurs on days you know that you'll be eating out.

Shake and Snack Options

Fortunately, this area of inquiry will be more fruitful than trying to cobble together a low carb meal at a fried chicken outlet. Many viable snack options can fit into a keto diet.

Firstly, consider canned fish. Sardines and mackerel are best for this purpose because they contain high amounts of fat. You can even include something like an avocado with a tin can of fish for a complete lunch. Tuna can be added if the amount of protein in the can is noted as part of your daily intake, and it's consumed with a large amount of fat. You can also get your fat from other sources like cheese, but don't eat the tuna by itself. Anchovies are also good as they are a low calorie but high fat fish, but note the salt content.

Speaking of cheese, it makes a great snack that can be incorporated into a keto diet. There are many kinds of cheese that you can consume including mozzarella cheese sticks, brie, or cheddar. Before consuming cheese be sure to check the nutrition facts to avoid any "hidden" problems. Avoid high protein consumption and any latent carbs.

Next, on the snack list are nuts. This has to be done with care and should be done after an initial "induction" phase in your diet. Macadamia nuts are the preferred choice as they are high fat and low protein. A one-ounce serving is 204 calories with only 2.2 grams of protein. You can consume other kinds of nuts, but you should be aware of the protein and carbs they contain. Nuts are high fiber, so for most varieties net carbs will be low, except for cashews. Try buying snack packs so that you can track the exact number of grams of protein.

Other snacks can be used as well. This includes prosciutto and panino along with deli meats. Keep in mind, however, that your consumption of these foods should be limited. Some contain hidden carbs and, in all cases, you want to track your protein consumption carefully. Eating a high protein meal without accompanying fat will be a problem.

Guacamole is a good snack food to consider, as are avocados in general.

Conclusion

If you're looking for an easy way to lose weight and feel better without having to experience deprivation, the keto diet might be for you. With the keto diet, you can enjoy rich and satisfying foods while still losing weight.

The keto diet is based on a few simple principles. We call the state of burning ketones (fat) for energy ketosis. Getting into ketosis is the first task faced when adopting a keto lifestyle.

First, limit your daily carbohydrate consumption to 20-30 grams per day. Second, define your protein consumption by matching grams consumed to your body mass. The rule to use is to eat at least 0.45 grams of protein per pound of body weight, but don't consume more than 0.5 grams of protein per pound of body weight. It's important not to consume too much protein because then the body will make protein into sugar, raising your blood sugar and defeating ketosis.

After you've planned out your protein and carbohydrates, eat fat. You can eat all the fat you want as long as you're not doing it to excess. But unlike Weight Watchers or other diet plans, you don't need to measure fat or count calories. Simply let your body tell you when you've had enough. If you eat fat until your satiated, then you won't have problems consuming too many calories. If you eat and still feel like you need to eat more – do it. Many beginners on keto get into trouble when they don't eat enough fat.

Keto has many health benefits. These include: losing weight, improved cholesterol, reduced blood sugar, lower triglycerides, and lower insulin levels. Keto can be very helpful for people with pre-diabetes or diabetics, but people on medication should discuss with their doctor first.

Fasting can be incorporated into the keto diet, if it's done correctly. Try out one of the intermittent fasting techniques to help accelerate and maintain weight loss after you're adapted to keto.

Electronic monitors can be very helpful to keep track of your progress at home. If you can afford it, you should get a blood sugar monitor and a ketone monitor. Track your fasting blood sugars and keep track of your ketones, ensuring that they fall within the 1.5-3.0 mmol/dL range. Also, you may want to track your HDL and triglycerides. Home monitors can be used to do this as well, allowing you to monitor progress more frequently and avoid unnecessary trips to the doctor's office.

Lastly, remember to keep a journal. It's important to keep track of your progress and helps you note not only how your triglycerides may be improving, but if you write down what you actually eat and find out you're not losing weight, it will make it easier to pinpoint problem areas where you can improve. One common mistake is people often consume too much protein and don't adjust their protein levels downward when they start losing weight.

Well, that does it for the book. I want to thank you for reading and hope that you found the book informative and that it will help you excel on your keto journey. If you've enjoyed the book, a review on Amazon would be much appreciated!

Bonus: Shopping list ideas

Building up your cabinet to serve keto compliant meals isn't all that difficult, but beginners often have trouble coming up with a complete shopping list. Here are some ideas to help get you started. The ingredients on this list can be used to make the recipes included in this book.

Produce
Baby spinach 1 pound
Cucumber 1
Bell pepper 1
Tomato 5
Cherry tomatoes 1 pint
Cabbage 1 head
White onions 3
Red onion 1
Green onion 1 bunch
Leeks 2 qty
Zucchini 2
Celery 1 stalk
Parsley 1 bunch
Cilantro 1 bunch
Basil 1 bunch
Garlic 2 heads
Avocados 4
Lemons 3
Limes 1
Jalapenos 2
Sliced mushrooms 15 ounces
Broccoli
Cauliflower
Asparagus

Pantry

Extra virgin olive oil
Anchovies
Green pesto
Tomato paste 1 tube
Tomato sauce 7 ounces
Kosher salt
Pepper
Chili powder
Cumin
Onion powder
Garlic powder
Paprika
Italian seasoning
Crushed red pepper flakes
Oregano
Dried minced onions
Dried parsley
Bone broth/stock 5 cups
Mayonnaise
Coconut aminos
Kalamata olives 1 jar
Walnuts or pecans ½ cup
Ground psyllium husk powder
Canned sardines
Canned mackerel (try canned in olive oil, better flavor)
Canned tuna
Coconut oil

Frozen

Riced cauliflower 10 ounces
Chicken wings (opt for low carb varieties, avoid honey barbecue)

Refrigerated/Dairy

Eggs 25 qty
Butter 1.75 pound (if you can, opt for butter from grass-fed cows)
Parmesan cheese, shredded
Ricotta cheese 2/3 cups
Cheddar cheese, shredded 4 cups
Gruyere cheese (3 ounces)
Cottage cheese 7 ounces
Goat cheese 8 ounces
Brie cheese 5 ounces
Heavy whipping cream
Coconut cream

Meat/Butcher

Grass fed ground beef 1.75 pounds
Minute steaks (8 qty)
Boneless or bone-in beef short ribs 2 pounds
Wild caught smoked salmon 12 ounces
Boneless chicken breast 1.75 pounds
Boneless thin pork chops 4 qty
Bone in chicken thighs 6 qty
Lamb chops 8 qty
Chorizo, 1 pound
Bacon 12 ounces
Pork loin
Pork sirloin steaks
Sea bass
Fresh sardines
Sausage (check carb content)
Rib eye steaks
Lamb –leg of lamb, shoulder and leg steaks

Deli and snacks
Ham 9 ounces
Sliced turkey
Prosciutto
Cheese sticks

Beverages
Red wine
White wine
Coffee
Tea
Bottled water
Soda water

Intermittent Fasting:

Eat what you love, heal your body, and improve your health through this secret weight loss guide! Living an healthy lifestyle, burn fat, and losing pounds at the same time has never been so simple! (Beginners friendly)

By Serena Baker

Foreword

For anyone seeking a boost into health or a bit of assistance losing some pesky weight—for anyone hoping to find renewed energy or better weight maintenance—for anyone struggling with food, strength, nutrition, or overall health, this book is made just for you.

Intermittent Fasting: Eat what you love, heal your body, and improve your health through this secret weight loss guide! Living an healthy lifestyle, burn fat, and losing pounds at the same time has never been so simple! Is a project I've been working on for a while, and I congratulate you for downloading it now as it has reached its perfection and completion. In this book, I aim to bring my education, experiences, and passions together to help readers reach all their fitness, dietary, and healthy goals.

My name is Serena Baker, and I graduated a few years ago with a bachelor's degree in Nutrition. I have been working since then to compile health and fitness books for anyone devoted on the path to personal growth. In this book specifically, my passion for fitness focuses on healthy diet and lifestyle first and foremost. I practice Intermittent Fasting in my own life and see consistent results regarding overall health, weight maintenance, and hunger level. So, I'm eager to share some tips of the trade with you. I'm excited to help as many people as I possibly can.

The chapters in this book will touch on everything about Intermittent Fasting, from the history of IF to the science behind it. The hard and fast facts, helpful recipes, ways to troubleshoot any issues, the different methods to try, ways to avoid hardship, and so much more. By the end of this book, you should find that you're confident about what IF is as well as what it will do for you once you start practicing it in your life, and you should have a plan set out to be able to do just that.

While many different books with this focus are available for a download, you've chosen this one, and I am both grateful and excited for you. Thank you for choosing this one, and I hope you look forward to all the good changes that are sure to be coming your way once you embrace Intermittent Fasting for yourself. Congratulations again, and good luck!

Introduction: The History of Intermittent Fasting

Within the past few years, the concept of Intermittent Fasting has started to trend heavily, impacting anyone interested in dieting and healthy living. Its origins, however, are much more ancient than most of us would ever think. In this chapter, you'll be introduced to the long history of Intermittent Fasting so that you can better understand how that trajectory leads to today. By the end of this section, you should feel confident that you know where the tradition came from, as well as what it has to do with you—reading this book in this very moment.

IF for Primitive Humans

Intermittent Fasting has been a practice as long as humans have existed. In the times of our most primitive ancestors, IF wasn't so much a chosen lifestyle as it was a necessity. It came down to the prevalence and availability of food—and the hunter's and gatherer's abilities to acquire it.

In these ancient times, people would have had to go longer between meals and sometimes perhaps spend days without eating. However, what arose from necessity produced incredible and even sustainable physical, mental, and emotional effects. These ancient people would have also (likely unintentionally) been able to concentrate better, live longer, slowing age and digest with ease consistently.

Primitive humans would also occasionally fast for shared purposes once societies and civilizations started assembling. For instance, before going off to war, communities would fast, and young people coming-of-age would fast as part of those rituals. Sometimes societies would also demand a fast as an offering to the gods or to implore the end of natural disasters such as floods or famines.

Religious Instances of IF

On the same vein as using a fast as an offering to the gods, many ancient cultures eventually required some fasting for their religion purposes. Consider Christianity. Orthodox Christians of the Greek variety still practice their ancient fasts, which comprise almost 200 days out of the year. Non-Orthodox Christians are also invited to fast whenever moved to do so to become closer to the Holy Trinity.

Consider Buddhism. The practice of intermittent fasting has always been essential to reaching enlightenment, because it helps the soul undo its ropes to the body. The enlightened one, Siddhartha, practiced fasting for many years as a method to acquire wisdom.

Consider Judaism. The day before Passover, it is an ancient tradition followed still today that the first-born child of each family should fast to celebrate the miracle from Moses' time that spared all Hebrew first-borns. Furthermore, Jewish people are invited to fast throughout the year at any point to celebrate a life lost, to appeal to God or a prophet, or to express sorrow for a sin or wrong committed.

Consider Islam. The holy month of Ramadan features a 4-week-long fast from the time the sun rises to the time the sun sets. During this time, drinks are also shunned, as well as alcohol drinking, smoking, or performing any bad habits or repetitive practices that don't serve the soul. Muhammad, the prophet of Islam, also suggested his followers fast every Monday and Thursday (essentially the 5:2 method, which we'll address in chapter 6!), but it's unclear how consistently this suggestion is heeded.

Other religions across the world have also required a temporary fast for spiritual reasons, and it is true that many have gotten closer to their gods through this practice. However, there are so many more benefits to fasting than just these spiritual ones, and these other applications are made clear in the next chapters.

From the Past to Now

On top of being used for survival and religious purposes, intermittent fasting has gained appeal through time for its medical applications as well. Even millennia before its trending popularity today, back in 400 BC, intermittent fasting made an appearance and gained popularity by the suggestion of Hippocrates.

Yes, *that* Hippocrates! The infamous "father of modern medicine" advocated for fasting to heal almost any internal injury or state of disease. He once wrote, "To eat when you are sick, is to feed your illness," if that gives you any indication of the incredible uses he found for the practice.

Other ancient Greek philosophers, writers, and historians have echoed these concepts from Hippocrates through time into the early years, AD. Essentially, just like how animals seem to "fast" when they're getting sick or feeling unwell, humans have the same instincts but often ignore them, pushing through the illness and feeding it with food when the body needs the exact opposite.

Past the ancient Greeks, however, other thinkers across time have affirmed the same feelings. For example, Paracelsus (another founder of modern medicine) famously wrote, "Fasting is the greatest remedy," and Benjamin Franklin (one of America's founding fathers) also once inscribed in a journal, "The best of all medicines is resting and fasting."

In the past, fasting has also been used as a form of political protest, and the most famous instance of this happening occurred with Mahatma Gandhi, who lasted 21 days at his longest period of fasting. His goals were to protest against India's dependence on Britain and to acquire freedom and integrity for his people. Many others have taken up fasting for similar aims, but none have been so successful or so famous, it seems.

Contemporary Applications

Now, it seems that fasting has gained new fame in the form of Intermittent Fasting, and the capital letters here are used intentionally to connote the almost "patented" application of these ancient theories in relation to health and weight loss in recent times.

This practice of Intermittent Fasting has been trending for the past few years, and its impact has spread widely since then. People have lost incredible amounts of weight. They've seen their energy levels improve drastically. They've been able to heal brain disorders and reverse the signs of aging. People across the world have come to understand what amazing uses fasting can have, and they are becoming healthier because of these realizations.

Doctors who have practiced fasting cures for decades have almost consistently welcomed the increased interest in IF these days, for they know how much good this practice can do for so many. Fasting is still used for religious and spiritual purposes, and some still practice it as they strive to survive. For others, IF today is revered as the so-called "fountain of youth," and many dietary plans are starting to incorporate its themes.

Overall, it seems that IF has been used throughout time for three main things: survival, spiritual connection, and body/mind health. These applications are valid today, but the focus tends toward that final point in the list: body/mind health. For those seeking a state of internal balance, IF can be a blessing. For those intrigued by IF, keep reading to find out more and to learn how to build this practice into your daily routine.

Chapter 1: Explaining Intermittent Fasting

What is Intermittent Fasting about after all, and how the heck does it work? This chapter will answer these questions and more. By the end of it, you should have a solid grasp on the practice of Intermittent Fasting, and you should also have a sense of why it's trending so much these days (as well as whether or not it sounds right for you).

What it Is

Intermittent Fasting is essentially the practice of restricting mealtimes, reducing snacking, or cutting out days of eating, based on the method one chooses. One of the most popular IF methods is 5:2, which is to eat five days a week and fast the other two. Others focus on eating windows and fasting periods within each day. The easiest method to start with for IF, however, is just to stop eating snacks.

So many of us snack unconsciously or when we're getting moody without any real hunger. So many of us eat unconsciously in general, and then we're confused why our bodies are holding onto the weight. Intermittent Fasting reminds the body what food is for, and it restarts that nutritional absorption potential. All you have to do is cut out the snacks, fast a few hours a day, or just drink water a few days a week.

IF is both a dietary choice and a lifestyle, but those who have the most success with IF will tell you that it became a lifestyle for them almost instantly. Sure, dieting plans and IF can match up nicely, but for some, IF requires no dietary change whatsoever. The point is to eat less and to eat less often. The brain and the body will respond in no time.

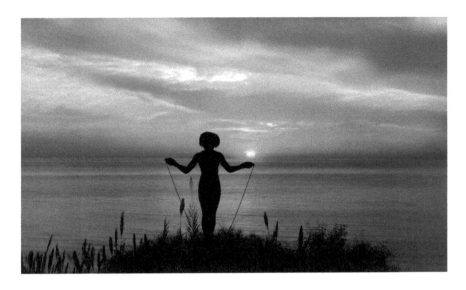

How it Works

There is a lot of science behind why IF works, and that will be detailed in chapter 4, but for now, it will suffice to say that IF works because it restricts the body of toxins and allows itself to clear out any excess. It gives the body a break and provides a moment to recalibrate, basically. And with this recalibration, neurotransmitters are released easier in the brain, and one's senses of hungry and full are adjusted back to how they should be. Once the food is eaten after the fast, too, nutritional absorption is boosted throughout the entire body, to the benefit of all one's organs.

Additionally, Intermittent Fasting recalibrates one's hormones in relation to stress and hunger so that balanced mood, patience, and intellect can be increased despite the seeming lack of food. IF tells the brain and body to restart. It makes your system go back to basics and clean out any gunk, and a lot of that gunk tends to be stored fat or water weight. It sees the toxins in your body and refuses to let you hold onto them. Overall, IF proves that a change in routine can have great and lasting effects on one's health.

Why People Start

People most often start Intermittent Fasting because they're interested in losing that pesky and lingering weight. They're trying to lose the holiday pounds, or they're interested in slimming down for beach season. Others are trying to let go of tens, if not hundreds, of pounds through this lifestyle shift. Basically, people most often start due to weight.

On the other hand, people have been known to start IF for the sake of reversing aging, healing the heart, or healing the brain. These effects will be detailed further in chapter 11! But for now, simply know that IF can restart a lot of systems in the body, not just the digestive and endocrine systems. IF can affect the hormones that contribute to aging, the ease with which blood flows through one's veins and arteries, and the potential for the brain to heal itself with increased plasticity.

As one final point, some people start IF because they're not satisfied with the bodies they're working to sculpt at the gym. Sometimes, people aren't particularly heavy, they're just hefty, and they're working on slimming down in the right places and bulking up in others. For these people, IF can help to repurpose lingering fat to either be burned for energy, or turned to muscle.

Why People Stay

People *start* Intermittent Fasting for a variety of reasons, but they always *stay* for the same reason, which is that the effects are undeniable and incredible. Regardless of why you start, you will stay because you will see changes in your body that you like, appreciate, and value. You will stay because you will have proven yourself strong in many ways and you will undoubtedly like what you've learned about yourself.

You will stay because IF will have helped you grow in ways you never imagined. Whether your goals were weight loss, anti-aging effects, sharper cognition, better memory, less disease, or otherwise, you will surely see that Intermittent Fasting can turn things around. All you need to do is devote some determination, a pinch of commitment, and a good lot of will power to the cause. Then, the sky's the limit, and your health is well within reach.

Chapter 2: Getting to the Facts

Before you know whether or not Intermittent Fasting will be right for you, it helps to go through the common myths, mistakes, and side-effects associated with this dietary choice and lifestyle. This chapter will do exactly that for you, and by the end, you should have most (if not all) of your concerns addressed.

8 Myths about IF Busted

There's a lot of misinformation circulating about Intermittent Fasting, but the truth is out there, too! Here are 8 myths about Intermittent Fasting and their respective *realities*.

1. MYTH: <u>Your body will definitely enter in starvation mode</u>.

    BUSTED: Your body will *not* definitely enter in starvation mode through Intermittent Fasting. Skipping meals or adjusting to longer periods between meals where you don't eat is not going to make you starve. It's going to help your body remember how to absorb nutrients. It's going to help you thrive instead.

2. MYTH: <u>You'll lose muscle in this endeavor</u>.

    BUSTED: This myth goes along the same lines as the first one, above. Just like your body won't enter the starvation mode (unless something goes very, very wrong or you're trying to do too much); your body won't lose muscle through IF. The only reason why IF *would* cause muscle loss would be if it was causing you to starve, but once again, the first myth addresses this falsity, making this myth false as well.

3. MYTH: <u>You'll almost assuredly overeat during eating windows, and that's not healthy at all</u>.

    BUSTED: While some people will have the *instinct* to overeat during eating windows, not everyone will overeat. Even those who do at the start will realize how to move forward without this overeating instinct in the future. Your body will urge you to overeat because, at the start, it won't realize what you're doing to it, but as long as you keep portion sizes largely the same and don't gorge on snacks, your body will adjust and so will your appetite.

4. MYTH: <u>Your metabolism will slow down dangerously</u>.

    BUSTED: This myth is also addressed in chapter 12's Questions & Answers, but the point is that your metabolism won't slow down just because you're eating less often. People who think this myth is true, only assume that restricted caloric intake will make one's metabolism slow down over time, but these individuals forget that IF isn't *necessarily* about cutting down calories overall (although methods like 20:4 don't leave much room for full caloric intake). It's actually about cutting down the *times* during which one consumes calories. There needn't be any caloric restriction whatsoever! It just depends on the practitioner and what he or she decides to do with dieting in addition to IF.

5. MYTH: <u>You'll only *gain* weight if you try skipping meals</u>.

BUSTED: This myth is based on the same logic that drives myth #3 about overeating. If you gorge yourself during your eating windows, you'll surely gain weight, but hardly anyone will continuously gorge with IF. Anyone who tries will realize how unsuccessful it is, so he or she will not *continuously* gorge in response. Anyone who doesn't realize his or her efforts with eating are unsuccessful will soon realize that something's wrong, as his or her weight shows no improvement. Skipping meals never *necessarily* means that someone will gain weight. It just means that people who skip meals *and gorge or overeat* when it *is* mealtime won't see the desired effects.

6.   MYTH: <u>During fast periods, you literally can't eat anything</u>.

BUSTED: This myth is partially true and partially false. It's true only for methods like 12:12, 14:10, 16:8, and 20:4 that require fasting and eating in alternation within each individual day. For 12:12 method, for example, you'd spend 12 hours fasting and 12 hours eating. In this case, you would definitely not eat anything or consume any calories during that 12-hour fasting window, but the same isn't true for methods that alternate between days "on" and days "off" between fasting and eating. For those types of methods, you absolutely can eat during fasting periods! It might feel counterintuitive as you read these words, but you don't explicitly have to eat *nothing* during fast periods. Most methods that have full days of fasting actually allow for caloric intake as long as it's restricted by 20-25% of one's normal intake. Therefore, for methods like 5:2, alternate-day, eat-stop-eat, and crescendo, on days when you're fasting, you can still consume around 500 calories, and that will help a lot!

7. MYTH: <u>There's only one way to do IF that's right and truly the best</u>.

BUSTED: This myth is absolutely and utterly false. There is no one right way to practice Intermittent Fasting, and part of the beauty of IF is that there *are* so many different methods, meaning each approaching IF likely has a few different options to choose from. Similarly, different body and personality types will be drawn to different methods, based on individuals' abilities and goals. IF is about flexibility, adjustment, and self-correction. There's no one right method for everyone, and there's no "best" method to strive for. Do whatever method feels right and suits your life, and once you've found it, practice it as long as you can! That's far more realistic and accessible.

8. MYTH: <u>It's not natural to fast like that</u>.

BUSTED: It's more natural to practice Intermittent Fasting than it is to eat three full meals each day! It's more connected to our evolutionary drives and to our primitive selves to eat like this. And it's better for our brains, hearts, cells, and digestive systems to have a break from food once in a while to recalibrate. As you learned in the Introduction, people have been practicing Intermittent Fasting as long as humans have been in existence. It's only myths like this that circulate today that make it seem like IF is foreign, unhealthy, and dangerous. Animals of all types become healthier after periods of fasting, and humans are no different. Remember that we are animals and that IF is in our nature. Proceed with that confidence and knowledge!

4 Most Common Mistakes & How to Avoid Them

Given the number of people who have tried Intermittent Fasting, there's no reason why you should have to suffer through the most common mistakes! Here are 4 of the most common mistakes and how to properly avoid them.

1. Make sure you're breaking fast correctly! Many people make the mistake of breaking fast with something high in calories or with a really big serving or a portion of their favorite food. However, breaking fast should be a thoughtful and almost meditative event that's not about gorging, feeling full, or rushing to eat. Breaking fast, especially if it's been a long time since you've eaten, should be slow and respectful, to both the food and to your body. Don't cram in the calories or eat a lot right away! Your body doesn't want *or need* that type of treatment. Start with a small something or eat slowly through a big portion, so that your body can adjust without cramps or aches and pains. Be thoughtful and don't rush to avoid this common mistake.

2. Make sure you don't waste your eating window! Some people turn to Intermittent Fasting because their days are hectic already and it makes sense not to eat all the time. Sometimes, people choose small eating windows, particularly because they don't normally eat a lot each day, to begin with. For people who make these sorts of choices especially, please be careful to don't waste valuable eating time! It might seem like you can work forever and push off eating until later and later and later, but sometimes, you could push it off until the eating window is totally gone, and your body certainly won't thank you for that. Be mindful of your timing and of when you're supposed to eat. Respect that allotment of time for what it can give to your body: health, nourishment, and energy.

3. <u>Make sure you don't try too much at once</u>! Some people try to fast while dieting while seriously exercising, and they wonder why they have no energy left! People who *want* to live high-intensity lifestyles like this are best suited toward plans like 5:2 (making sure not to exercise on those two fast days!). But even so, these individuals shouldn't put their bodies through *too much* stress with the addition of Intermittent Fasting. If you are attempting to do all three (diet, fast, and exercise), and you notice your energy level dropping, your mood swinging, or your belly burning, it might be time to cut back on one of those elements. Do a little less exercise! Eat a little more when you can! Try to add in some more calories! IF isn't about starvation, and it should never lead to that when done correctly and with healthy intentions. Remember that as you proceed with your journey.

4. <u>Make sure you don't give up too soon</u>! It's often the case that people give up on IF before the first week is over. They're frustrated by these feelings of hunger, and they feel convinced they'll never see results. Don't be duped into this way of thinking! Remember the power of your will. Be stubborn! Push through that first week and look forward to seeing results. They sometimes aren't as immediate as you'd hope, but that doesn't mean they're not coming! Even if you can tell the method you chose isn't working, try to last out the first week before troubleshooting and choosing a different one. For people who aren't convinced even after switching methods, try to go a whole two weeks before giving up entirely. You never know—it could be that last day in two weeks that your body starts to show results! Keep a focused mindset and a clear eye on your goals. Push through any hardship and be stubborn with your hopes and actions! Success will come in time.

6 Unexpected Side-Effects of IF

Some of the side-effects of Intermittent Fasting are easily assumed, but some are far more unexpected. This section details six of the most commonly unexpected side-effects associated with the practice.

1. Irritability is one of the most commonly unexpected side-effects from Intermittent Fasting, but it is very prevalent, especially for people just beginning to transition into the lifestyle. People get angry! It's a thing. People get snippy and sassy when they're waiting for food. Unfortunately, this will be you, but you're definitely going to learn a lot about yourself during this period, and you'll eventually grow *through* these irritable feelings. Be patient with yourself (and especially patient with others). The irritability will fade, I promise.

2. Feeling cold is another of those things none of us would likely expect about from practicing Intermittent Fasting (or maybe it is, and I'm just off on this one!). You will probably feel extra sensitive to the cold through your fingers and toes while you're fasting, but this side-effect is totally normal! Don't be alarmed when you feel it. Instead, just know that it means your body is burning fat and your blood sugar is decreasing, and these effects are standard and healthy to experience. Drink a little extra hot tea or wear a few extra layers to help keep warm.

3. Heartburn is a more uncommon side-effect of Intermittent Fasting, but it's another thing that's totally natural. Your stomach is used to producing acids to digest the foods you're consuming, and when you start adjusting to IF, these acids are being produced at times when you're potentially fasting, causing heartburn or reflux issues. With time, this side-effect should be mitigated if not totally alleviated. Keep drinking water and try not to eat foods that are

super greasy or spicy when you do breakfast. If things don't get better, consider speaking with your doctor or nutritionist.

4. Bloating is a side-effect related to #5 below, Constipation. When you transition into Intermittent Fasting, your stomach is going to be processing things in a way that it hasn't in a long, long time—possibly ever. There will be weird side-effects like this for some, but it's all part of that adjustment period, and these issues should resolve themselves in a week or so. Drink a lot of water to aid the situation!

5. Constipation is related to Bloating, and it's just one of those things that might happen in your body as you get used to eating less or at incredibly different times than normal. Remember to drink a lot of water so whatever *is* in your system has enough hydration to come out without stress. Within a few weeks, the water cure (drink A LOT!!!) should help flush out the issue.

6. More frequent urination is common as well, and this situation most often arises due to the displacement of eating for the sake of the fast. During these fast periods, individuals are invited to drink anything (that doesn't have too many calories), and this often translates to a full bladder almost constantly—at least in the beginning! When things get tough, you'll want to drink more water. If things get gurgle-y or constipated on the inside, you'll want to drink more water. If you have headaches or get lightheaded, you'll want some water with a pinch of salt. If you need energy, you'll grab the coffee. You get the picture. Expect frequent bathroom runs.

Chapter 3: Benefits of Intermittent Fasting

There are so many incredible benefits possible for you once you choose Intermittent Fasting, and this chapter is dedicated to those individual benefits. First, we will go through 20 general positive points that arise from Intermittent Fasting, and then we will address five specific benefits each, for women and then for men, respectively. At the end of this section, you should feel excited by all the possibilities provided by IF, and you should be much better able to tell whether or not this lifestyle is right for you.

20 General Benefits

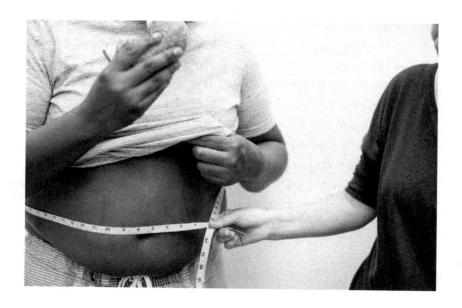

Intermittent Fasting has such incredible potential for so many different body and personality types, and 20 of the coolest benefits are listed below.

1. Incredible weight loss potential

2. Lowered insulin & blood sugar levels

3. Increased preservation of muscle mass

4. Increased neuroplasticity

5. Cancer healing potential

6. Lower blood pressure

7. Lower cholesterol

8. Overall longer life

9. Restructured nutrition absorption potential

10. Overall increased feeling of well-being

11. More energy for more tasks and activities

12. Improved cognition and mental processing

13. Better memory access and potential

14. Increased sense of welfare

15. High degree of independence and autonomy in choosing one's strategy or method

16. Overall ease in starting and maintaining one's approach

17. Increased (sense of) will power

18. Better ability to tune in with one's body

19. Increased awareness of the effects of food on the body, mind, and emotions

20. Ability to eat the same things and still lose weight

5 Benefits for Women in Specific

For women specifically, Intermittent Fasting poses certain trials and opportunities. Here are 5 of the most exciting benefits women can expect to see.

1. Lessened period cramps

2. Regulated or relieved process of menstruation

3. The potential for restricted fertility (this is a benefit for some!) at least during fast periods

4. Reduced internal inflammation that would lead to cancers of the reproductive organs

5. Better hormone regulation and healthier production

5 Benefits for Men in Specific

For men specifically, Intermittent Fasting can do a few different things than it can for women, and 5 of the best benefits are listed below.

1. Increased testosterone levels

2. Reduction of lingering estrogen levels from foods

3. Increases HGH (the Human Growth Hormone)

4. Reduced internal inflammation that would lead to prostate or renal cancer

5. Increased virility and sexual stamina overall

Chapter 4: The Science of Intermittent Fasting

You've learned a lot about Intermittent Fasting so far, but you still likely don't understand *why* it all works so well for dieting and health. This chapter is the antidote to that confusion! You will learn how Intermittent Fasting affect the body, how it interacts with diabetes, heart health, aging, and finally, the female body. By the end of this chapter, you should feel both highly informed about IF and aware of a few potential complications.

How IF Affects the Body

When you're feeling hungry, your body is under the sway of two very important hormones: leptin and ghrelin, and Intermittent Fasting affects both of those hormones substantially. In a typical situation, leptin decreases sensations of being hungry, and ghrelin makes you feel hungry instead. While leptin is secreted from fat cells throughout the body, ghrelin is only secreted from the stomach's lining. Together, leptin and ghrelin communicate with the brain's hypothalamus, telling the body when to stop or start eating. During IF, these hormones are released less often, causing the body to have a whole different experience of hunger and fullness.

Another important hormone in the context of eating and hunger suppression is insulin itself. The pancreas produces insulin, and it regulates how much glucose exists in our blood. Ultimately, high or low amounts of insulin affect the individual's weight greatly. Too little insulin and one can't keep weight on. Too much insulin and one can't lose weight whatsoever. While it seems that lower insulin is desired, there has to be a healthy balance, for *too low* insulin is actually disastrous for the body since glucose (or blood sugar) is a large part of how the body gets energy.

One final influencer of the body's hunger and weight loss situation is the individual's thyroid. If the thyroid is overactive, metabolism will work quickly, and energy, health, and weight will be affected. Conversely, an underactive thyroid will slow metabolism, energy, and health, and it will contribute to increased weight.

In the end, Intermittent Fasting affects the individual's weight by varying the production of these three important hormones and by working with the thyroid's natural potential. Essentially, those practicing IF will trigger these hormones to be released less often (or more consistently if the person is obese or diabetic to start with) due to the less-frequent eating schedule. Eventually, even the thyroid's effects should become balanced out through this altered eating schedule.

IF and Diabetes

For people with diabetes, Intermittent Fasting poses certain risks as well as incredible benefits. People with diabetes have altered insulin levels compared to the non-diabetic person, due to insulin resistance in their bodies. People with Type 1 diabetes cannot make insulin. They need to take insulin daily to have the energy and vigor to live. People with Type 2 diabetes have bodies that don't produce much insulin or don't use that insulin well at all.

With these altered productions of insulin, the blood sugar levels of the body have no way to be regulated, meaning that there's more standing glucose in the blood at all times with no way for it to get into the cells to be used for natural and physical energy. This higher blood sugar level can cause additional problems for the individual over time, but there is no legitimate cure other than taking insulin daily.

Intermittent Fasting, however, can provide a temporary cure when applied correctly in the lives of diabetic individuals (whose diabetic conditions are not severe). When IF is done on a daily basis with just a few fasting hours a day, people with diabetes show improved weight, blood sugar levels, and standing glucose levels. These individuals are not recommended to skip entire meals or fast for days at a time. Also, is not recommended for these people to strictly diet while they're applying IF. Instead, it works better to make food portions smaller and to eat fewer snacks in between.

IF and Heart Health

Heart health is a complicated issue in today's world. We all want to be healthy and thrive, but the foods we eat and the activities we engage in often don't align with those goals, and those more immediate actions win out. In effect, many of our hearts aren't as healthy as they could be. Heart disease is still the biggest killer in the world to this day. However, the introduction of Intermittent Fasting into someone's lifestyle can greatly alter this potential, for it can reduce many risks associated with heart disease.

For example, recent studies done on animals have proved that the practice of Intermittent Fasting improves numerous risk factors for heart disease. Some of these improvements include lowered cholesterol, reduced inflammation in the body, balanced blood sugar levels, and lower blood pressure. Essentially, IF won't cure heart disease, but it will reduce several risk factors that may exist in one's body (with or without him or her knowing).

When it comes down to it, as long as one's Intermittent Fasting experience involves the reintroduction of electrolytes into the body, there's no potential harm posed to the heart whatsoever. There's only potential for growth, bolstering, and strengthening. However, without the right reintroduction of electrolytes, there *is* still the possibility of heart palpitations in individuals attempting IF. The heart needs electrolytes for its stability and efficacy, so as long as you drink a bit of salt with your water, your heart will only thank you!

IF and Aging

People love to talk about how Intermittent Fasting can reverse the effects of aging, and they're not wrong! The tricky part is elucidating the science behind the process they're referencing. The anti-aging potential tied up with Intermittent Fasting applies mostly to two things: 1) your brain and 2) your whole body, through what's called "autophagy."

Overall, Intermittent Fasting heals the body through its ability to rejuvenate the cells. With this restricted caloric intake due to eating schedule or timing, the body's cells can function with less limitation and confusion while producing more energy for the body to use. In effect, the cells function more efficiently while the body can burn more fat and take in more oxygen for the organs and blood, encouraging the individual to live longer with increased sensations of "youth."

About those two original examples, Intermittent Fasting has been proven 1) to keep the brain fit and agile. It improves overall cognitive function and memory capacity as well as cleverness, wit, and quick, clear thinking in the moment. Furthermore, Intermittent Fasting 2) keeps the cells fit and agile through autophagy (which is kickstarted by IF), where the cells are encouraged to clean themselves up and get rid of any "trash" that might be clogging up the works. By just restricting your eating schedule a little bit each day (or each week), you can find your brain power boosted and your body ready for anything.

IF and the Female Body

Intermittent Fasting requires a different technique than most diets do, which is why it's more often referred to as a lifestyle. Additionally, this variance means that the effects of IF on the female body are a little different than the effects of the standard diet. For instance, dieting will easily cause weight loss in most people, but IF is a little trickier and much less consistent for women especially.

The female body, being created with birthing potential, has specific needs that are altered through an Intermittent Fasting eating schedule. With less hormones being released (which tell women when they are hungry and full) there is less fat being stored in their bodies and less fertility when it comes to their later aims of reproducing. In combination with a strict diet that counts calories or restricts fats, Intermittent Fasting can be dangerous for women of all ages.

For women who still want to work with Intermittent Fasting, there's a lot of hope left for you! Just make sure to follow these four steps to ensure that you're doing it in the most healthy way for your body and your future children. First, make sure you're very connected to your body. You'll want to be very aware if something on the inside seems "off" or "wrong" (bodily, emotionally, and mentally), especially considering all that's at stake, hormonally and reproductively.

Second, make serious effort to be aware of your body's cycles and note when things go askew. Without the right awareness of your menstruation, you risk going a long time with an altered cycle. This alteration might not sound like a lot, but it can affect many different aspects of your body and your childrearing potential.

Third, please don't try to combine strict dieting and Intermittent Fasting. I know you want to be fit and strong and slim, but you still want to make sure you're getting enough fat and calories, considering what your body is able to do with these right amounts of fat and calories.

Fourth and finally, make sure you're also not exercising too ferociously while you first transition to Intermittent Fasting. If you've been trying IF as a lifestyle for a while, you're welcome to add fitness and exercise back into the mix, but it is really dangerous for the female body to combine two intense practices at once. I understand the urge to lose weight and be healthy, but you'll need to make sure you're not eliminating *too much* from your body at any given time.

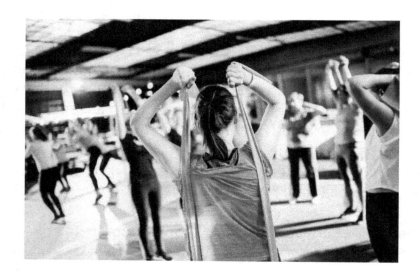

Given the complexity of the subject, I thought it was really useful to explain how Intermittent Fasting acts specifically on the female body. I dedicated a whole new book to it (*Intermittent Fasting for Women: Learn How You Can Use This Science to Support Your Hormones, Lose Weight, Enjoy Your Food, and Live a Healthy Life Without Suffering from Your Dietary Habits*)

If you're interested in the subject, I suggest you try to have a look at it. You can find the information here!

Chapter 5: For Some, Not Others

Given those potential complications concerning Intermittent Fasting, it is undeniable that it works perfectly for some, but not as well for others. This chapter will walk you through the body types and personality types that are well-suited for IF as well as those that are *definitely not* a good match. At the end of this section, you should know clearly whether or not IF is the next lifestyle choice for you.

5 Personality Types Perfect for IF

Some personality types are just perfectly matched for Intermittent Fasting, and 5 of them are included below.

1. <u>Sensitive introverts</u> are a great match for Intermittent Fasting. These types of people are often quiet and spend a lot of time alone, which means they're incidentally very in tune with the inner workings of their bodies and with the tendencies of their minds. By extension, therefore, these people will be extremely productive if they decide to try Intermittent Fasting because they'll be very aware of things going wrong almost immediately, but they'll also be very conscious of things going right.

2. <u>Problem solver</u> personalities will love the excitement provided by Intermittent Fasting! They'll see the problems posed by their bodies and their weight, and they'll be very eager to solve those problems with a combination of intelligence, cleverness, and bodily intuition. These people will meet the challenge of weight loss or boosting brain health with enthusiasm and determination, knowing that a solution is in sight. They will be very likely to succeed in all IF endeavors.

3. Health nut personalities will love Intermittent Fasting for its interesting and divergent approach to body and mind health. They will love the long history of IF, as well as the words of assurance from great minds like Hippocrates, Paracelsus, and Benjamin Franklin. They will be devoted to the task of learning and perfecting IF in their lives based on all this appreciation, too, for they will know that learning and perfecting IF means they'll be learning more about and perfecting the self to be as healthy and vibrant as possible.

4. Fitness experts will love the potential Intermittent Fasting has to reinvent their bodies completely. They will appreciate the logic behind IF, too, in that it comes from the most primitive and ancient humans' survival expressions. They will see IF as a method of living out constant fitness, and they will be encouraged to approach their workouts differently, based on what they can achieve with restricted eating times. Furthermore, fitness experts will be highly intrigued by IF, which will make them willing to try things out—at least until things prove detrimental (which they will find, they won't).

5. Confident and brave adventurers, both in general and regarding food, will appreciate what Intermittent Fasting has to offer as well. These adventurers will recognize that change (of approach and focus) is almost always productive so that they will be drawn to the IF experience like flies to food! These types of people will try IF likely because they want to prove they can do it, but they'll stick with the strategy because they'll feel elated after their bodies adjust to these odd and new eating times. They'll try it out for the adventure and stay for the blessings they receive.

5 Body Types Perfect for IF

Similarly, certain body types are spot-on in alignment with the goals and possibilities of Intermittent Fasting. 5 such body types are listed below.

1. <u>Heavy people</u> are bound to see huge successes in their attempts at Intermittent Fasting. As long as they can stay dedicated and committed to the eating and fasting time slots—and as long as they don't overeat during those eating windows—they should be able to see that fat almost melt away within weeks. In fact, heavy people who commit to Intermittent Fasting have the most to gain from their efforts, although they may have to add slight dieting or slight exercise to the mix to see these gains sooner.

2. <u>People with belly pudge</u> are also extremely well-suited to try Intermittent Fasting, for they should see results incredibly quickly. Just a bit of belly pudge mixed with a little less time spent eating each day can have a beautiful outcome, as long as the practitioner is dedicated and committed to his or her efforts. These types of people likely won't have to add diet or exercise to their routines to see that pudge disappear, but if they're interested in building muscle, they may have to add a little exercise after all.

3. <u>People with generally-fit bodies</u> pair well with the Intermittent Fasting lifestyle, too. These people are often already somewhat conscious of health, weight, and wellness. Additionally, they're often already conscious of how eating the right foods can act as a healing strategy for the body, mind, and soul. Therefore, these fit-bodied individuals won't have so much room to grow or change (bodily) with Intermittent Fasting, but they will find their mindsets and emotions changed in ways that are intriguing and lasting through this new lifestyle practice.

4. <u>People who are slim or heavy yet have trouble building muscle</u> are extremely well-suited to try Intermittent Fasting paired with light exercise. These types of people would do well with a method like 5:2 that requires five days of standard eating and exercise paired with two days in the week of fasting, wherein, for each day. No exercise is performed and only 500 calories are consumed. With the right alternation of eating and exercise with fasting and contemplation, these individuals are liable to see incredible growth of mind paired with an impressive loss of fat, favoring muscle.

5. <u>Women who are pear-shaped</u> have extra stores of body fat at the hips, tummy, and thighs, which makes them excellent candidates for great and lasting change through Intermittent Fasting! IF will help these women burn that fat into energy, and it will encourage their bodies to stop storing fat there in the future. With just a momentary recalibration through IF or a lifetime switch to the exercise, any pear-shaped woman can see those hips shrink down to a smaller size. With determination, commitment, and practice, any bodily circumstances can change.

5 Personality Types that Don't Work

It might sound harsh, but some personality types aren't well-suited for the practice and lifestyle of Intermittent Fasting. If you relate to any of the 5 personality types below, make sure to do a lot of searching before you decide to try IF for yourself.

1. <u>Obsessive health or fitness experts</u> will definitely enjoy what Intermittent Fasting can do for them or their fitness-related clients, but these people are not encouraged to get dedicated to IF as a lifestyle, for they are bound to lose far too much. These people are only at risk with IF because their personalities are *obsessive* in

nature. They won't be able to stop thinking about the fast, what it's doing for them, how to do it right, how to do it best, and how to be the best. These people are very likely to focus on the wrong parts of IF and turn it into an obsession rather than a healthy lifestyle. If anyone of this nature wants to try IF, I recommend they practice a little personality-softening (or ego-dampening) first.

2. <u>Compulsive athletes</u> are also potentially problematic about choosing Intermittent Fasting. If these types of people go the IF route, they're sure to see success, and they're sure to feel good, but it's very easy for compulsive athletes to push things *too far* for the sake of health or success. They can easily push way past their comfort zones without noticing, which is beneficial for sports, but it's not beneficial for one's body when the potential risk is one's health. For compulsive athletes who want to try IF still, I recommend spontaneous skipping method. These people are invited to take on the less intense strategies like this one to experience what IF has to offer without losing themselves (and their health) in the process.

3. <u>Overly-controlling people</u> *might* enjoy Intermittent Fasting, but they could easily get too stuck in the details to fully appreciate what's happening. These people are liable to get too obsessed with perfection or with forcing the process to produce results (when they're not immediate or obvious). It's easy that they push themselves too fast and too hard to see results. Ultimately, these people can certainly grow, personality-wise, through Intermittent Fasting, but I'm concerned that their bodies might not benefit if their minds get the better of them. For those who qualify as overly-controlling and still want to try IF, just be patient with yourself as much as possible, and try not to force any of the processes.

4. <u>Scatterbrained people and "space cadets"</u> are similar to overly-controlling people when it comes to Intermittent Fasting because they can grow a lot through IF, personality-wise, but their main downfall is very different from that of overly-controlling people.

191

Essentially, scatterbrained people or so-called "space cadets" often don't have the wherewithal to make sure they're sticking to schedules and following through on their IF timing goals. There's an obvious benefit to personalities like this, and some of my best friends qualify as "space cadets," but I'm not sure I'd recommend that they take on such a huge decision as trying IF—not unless they're truly ready to commit with full-force of body and mind.

5. Overly-anxious or worrisome people (as well as hypochondriacs) are not recommended to try Intermittent Fasting unless they're ready for some intense and serious personality work. These people are liable to get caught up in the details so much that they can't progress or move forward to be able to see real success with Intermittent Fasting. People who qualify as overly-anxious, worrisome, or hypochondriacs are still absolutely encouraged to *try* IF, but only as long as they're willing to work through the darkest parts of themselves first! Most people with these traits aren't ready for that, however, so I recommend they steer clear until they're emotionally and mentally better healed.

6 Body Types that Don't Work

Some body types, too, are simply not oriented to work well with Intermittent Fasting. It might not be what you want to hear, but if your body type correlates with any of the 6 below, you might want to take a step back and reevaluate before you decide to try IF.

1. People with body dysphoria are highly problematic candidates when it comes to Intermittent Fasting. These individuals receive false or skewed self-images through various means of perception, which means their sense of what's good about (or what needs to change about) themselves is absolutely off-kilter. These people may want to

try IF even though they're beautifully fit and healthy. They may force themselves to try harsher IF methods because they don't feel like they're seeing the right results yet. People with body dysphoria are encouraged to work on their self-image and accepting themselves before they try to change anything.

2. People with eating disorders are also incredibly problematic candidates for Intermittent Fasting. IF doesn't have to be practiced in unhealthy ways, and for the most part, it isn't. However, people with eating disorders (or with a history of them) will find that IF is an accidental gateway to a side of themselves that's not healthy whatsoever. People who are healing eating disorders are encouraged to try IF only with the verification from their doctors or nutritionists that this step is healthy and safe. Otherwise, wait a little while, heal yourself first, and then work on IF if your body can take it.

3. Overly-thin people probably don't need to try Intermittent Fasting at all. Most people apply IF to their lives to see weight loss, muscle building, or slimming progress. But people who are already very thin pose a threat to themselves and their health by adding IF to the mix. If you're already thin due to dieting, steer clear of IF. If you're thin due to exercise, cut the exercise if you want to try IF and make sure to keep eating the same number of calories! If you're thin due to genetics, it's debatable, but I still recommend you *not* try IF unless your doctor or nutritionist approves. You wouldn't want to do damage to yourself accidentally, would you!?

4. People with severe diabetes risk doing serious damage to their bodies and internal systems if they attempt Intermittent Fasting. If you severely have diabetes, IF might frustrate you because you won't be able to try it purely, and you will still have to take insulin throughout the process. It's essential to note that you *won't be able to heal diabetes with IF*. If that's your goal, turn away right now. For those who just wanted to try IF to help the situation, you might be a

little misled, too. People with severe diabetes should not try to restrict caloric intake seriously, they should not try to drink just liquids, and they should not try to fast for long periods; their bodies will not respond positively, and there are disastrous consequences. If people with severe diabetes still want to try IF, they're encouraged not to. Don't limit *when* you eat, eat healthier, more whole foods whenever possible.

5. <u>People with leaky gut</u> are not encouraged to turn to Intermittent Fasting to become healthier. In fact, people with leaky gut are often struggling to receive full nutrients from the foods they're actually consuming, so it's like they're on an IF lifestyle gone-wrong constantly, without even choosing it. Heal that leaky gut issue before trying IF, for the two together will put your body and health in a truly dangerous place.

6. <u>Pregnant & breastfeeding women</u> are not suggested to try Intermittent Fasting. There is much debate surrounding the issue of breastfeeding women, and it *can* be done safely, but for pregnant women, the case is not the same. The pregnant mother will be *unavoidably* providing nutrients to the child she's growing inside her, and if she restricts calories in any way, she will do damage to the fetus and its abilities to grow and develop. Divergently, breastfeeding mothers can supplement breastmilk with formula if things get tricky, and they can try less intensive IF methods to keep the breastmilk flowing well if they're really stuck to the idea of trying IF.

Chapter 6: The Many Faces of Intermittent Fasting

There are so many different ways to practice Intermittent Fasting that this entire chapter is dedicated to just those methods. I will walk you through 10 specific and different methods for IF before ending with a section on *how* to make your choice. By the end of this chapter, if you've chosen to try IF, you should feel that your IF plans have direction and form, and you should be excited to implement these new plans into your daily routine.

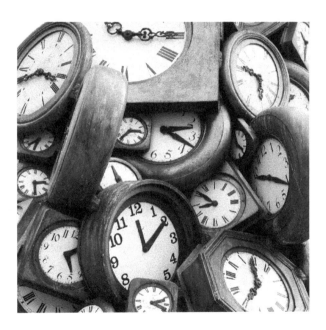

Explanation of Different Methods

Before you can start practicing Intermittent Fasting and incorporating it into your lifestyle, you'll have to know all the possibilities so you can choose the right one(s) for yourself, your goals, your habits, and your body/personality type. Read through the following 10 suggestions to find which methods sound most right to you.

Lean-Gains Method

The lean-gains method essentially focuses on the combined efforts of rigorous exercise, fasting, and a healthy diet. The fame surrounding this approach comes from its acclaimed success at turning fat directly into muscle. The goal is to fast within each day for 14-16 hours, starting when you wake up.

The ideal approach to lean-gains seems to be that you wake up and fast until 1 pm, doing some stretches and pre-workout warmups just before noon. Starting at noon, you would engage in training in whatever exercise you choose for an hour or less, ending with you breaking fast around 1 pm. Your meal at this time would be the largest of the day.

You would engage in your day as normal past then, as possible, eating again around 4 pm, then eating for the final time around 9 pm, giving yourself a ~15-hour fast until the next day at 1 pm. If you choose this approach yet feel a bit overwhelmed, you can work up to 15 hours, starting with a 13- or 14-hour fast only for the first week, building up to 15- or 16-hour fasting after that.

16:8 Method

16:8 method is one of the most popular methods among Intermittent Fasters. Essentially, you spend 16 hours within each day fasting, and the other 8 hours are your eating window. Most people try to choose their 8-hour eating window to be the times when they're primarily active. If you're a night person, feel free to make it a little later. Hold off eating during the daytime as much as possible then breakfast around 3 or 4 pm. For morning people, breakfast earlier, say, around 11 am, stopping food consumption by 7 pm.

16:8 is an incredibly flexible method that works for many different kinds of people. It's even flexible once you decide to try a particular fasting to eating window ratio. For example, if you don't seem to be jiving with the 11-7pm eating window, you can absolutely alter the next day to suit your needs better. Maybe try waiting until later in the day to breakfast! Try what you need to do, as long as you're keeping to that 16:8-hour ratio.

Whereas lean-gains method technically applies the same hourly ratio, it's much more strict regarding healthy diet and exercise regimen. 16:8 method does not need any type of exercise booster, but that's up to the practitioner. It is always best to try adding healthy dietary choices to one's IF eating schedule but don't try to restrict too many calories, as it can incorporate to feelings of lightheadedness and low energy. With 16:8, you can eat what you need and swap the hours around as desired.

14:10 Method

Similar to 16:8 method, 14:10 requires fasting and eating in varying degrees within each day. In this case, you would fast for 14 hours and engage in eating for a 10-hour window afterward. This method has the same flexibility as 16:8 in terms of what time of day it's arranged around, and how easy it is to troubleshoot. But it's additionally flexible in the sense that the eating window is two hours longer, accommodating people with more intense physical routines or daily demands, as well as people who simply need to eat a little later in the day to feel well.

20:4 Method

Whereas 14:10 method was an easier step *down* from 16:8 method, 20:4 method is definitely a step *up* in terms of difficulty. It's a more intense method certainly, for it requires 20 hours of fasting within each day with only a 4-hour eating window for the individual to gain all his or her nutrients and energy.

Most people who try this method end up having either one large meal with several snacks or they have two smaller meals with fewer snacks. 20:4 is flexible in that sense—the sense whereby the individual chooses how the eating window is divided amongst meals and snacks.

20:4 method is tricky, for many people instinctually over-eat during the eating window, but that's neither necessary nor is it healthy. People that choose 20:4 method should try to keep meal portions around the same size that they would normally have been without fasting. Experimenting on how many snacks are needed will be helpful as well with this method.

Many people end up working up to 20:4 from other methods, based on what their bodies can handle and what they're ready to attempt. Few start with 20:4, so if it's not working for you right away, please don't be too hard on yourself! Step it back to 16:8 and then see how soon you can get back to where you'd like to be.

The Warrior Method

The warrior method is quite similar to 20:4 method in that the individual fasts for 20 hours within each day and breaks fast for a 4-hour eating window. The difference is in the outlook and mindset of the practitioner, however. Essentially, the thought process behind warrior method is that, in ancient times, the hunter coming home from stalking prey or the warrior coming home from battle would really only get one meal each day. One meal would have to provide sustenance for the rest of the day, recuperative energy from the ordeal, and sustainable energy for the future.

Therefore, practitioners of warrior method are encouraged to have one large meal when they breakfast, and that meal should be jam-packed with fats, proteins, and carbs for the rest of the day (and for the days ahead). Just like with 20:4 method, however, it can sometimes be too intense for practitioners, and it's very easy to scale this one back in forcefulness by making up a method like 18:6 or 17:7. If it's not working, don't force it to work past two weeks, but do try to make it through a week to see if it's your stubbornness or if it's just a mismatch with the method.

12:12 Method

12:12 method is a little easier, along with the lines of 14:10, rather than 16:8 or 20:4. Beginners to Intermittent Fasting would do well to try this one right off the bat. Some people get 12 hours of sleep each night and can easily wake up from the fasting period, ready to engage with the eating window. Many people use this method in their lives without even knowing it.

To go about 12:12 method in your life, however, you'll want to be as purposeful about it as you can be. Make sure to be strict about your 12-hour cut-offs. Make sure it's working and feeling good in your body, and then you're invited to take things up a notch and try, say, 14:10 or maybe your own invention, like 15:11. As always, start with what works and then move up (or down) to what feels right (and even possibly *better*).

5:2 Method

5:2 method is popular among those who want to take things up a notch generally. Instead of fasting and eating within each day, these individuals take up a practice of fasting two whole days out of the week. The other 5 days are free to eat, exercise, or diet as desired, but those other two days (which can be consecutive or scattered throughout the week) must be strictly fasting days.

For those fasting days, it's not as if the individual can't eat anything altogether, however. In actuality, one is allowed to consume no more than 500 calories each day for this Intermittent Fasting method. I suppose these fasting days would be better referred to as "restricted-intake" days, for that is a more accurate description.

5:2 method is extremely rewarding, but it is also one of the more difficult ones to attempt. If you're having issues with this method, don't be afraid to experiment the next week with a method like 14:10 or 16:8, where you're fasting and eating within each day. If that works better for you, don't be ashamed to embrace it! However, if you're dedicated to having days "on" and days "off" with fasting and eating, there are other alternatives, too.

Eat-Stop-Eat (24-Hour) Method

The eat-stop-eat or 24-hour method is another option for people who want to have days "on" and "off" between fasting and eating. It's a little less intense than 5:2 method, and it's much more flexible for the individual, based on what he or she needs. For instance, if you need a literal 24-hour fast each week and that's it, you can do that. On the other hand, if you want a more flexible 5:2 method-type thing to happen, you can work with what you want and create a method surrounding those desires and goals.

The most successful approaches to the eat-stop-eat method have involved more strict dieting (or at the very least, cautious and healthy eating) during the 5 or 6 days when the individual engages in the week's free-eating window. For the individual to truly see success with weight loss, there will have to be some caloric restriction (or high nutrition focus) those 5 or 6 days, too, so that the body will have a version of consistency in health and nutrition content.

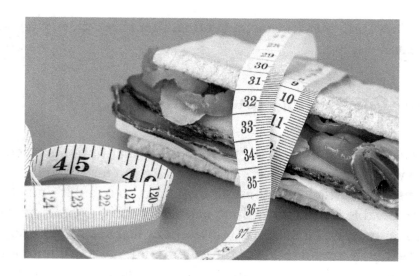

On the one or two days each week the individual decides to fast, there can still be highly-restricted caloric intake. As with 5:2 method, he or she can consume no more than 500 calories worth of food and drink during these fasting days so that the body can maintain energy flow and more.

If the individual engages in exercise, those workout days should absolutely be reserved for the 5 or 6 free-eating days. The same goes for 5:2 method. Try not to exercise (at least not excessively) on those days that are chosen for fasting. Your body will not appreciate the added stress when you're taking in so few calories. As always, you can choose to move up from eat-stop-eat to another method if this works easily and you're interested in something more. Furthermore, you can start with a strict 24-hour method and then move up to a more flexible eat-stop-eat approach! Do what feels right, and never be afraid to troubleshoot one method for the sake of choosing another.

Alternate-Day Method

The alternate-day method is similar to eat-stop-eat and 5:2 methods because it focuses on individual days "on" and "off" for fasting and eating. The difference for this method, in particular, is that it ends up being at least 2 days a week fasting, and sometimes, it can be as many as 4.

Some people follow very strict approaches to alternate-day method and literally fast every other day, only consuming 500 calories or less on those days designated for fasting. Some people, on the other hand, are much more flexible, and they tend to go for two days eating, one day fasting, two days eating, one day fasting, etc. The alternate-day method is even more flexible than eat-stop-eat in that sense, for it allows the individual to choose how he or she alternates between eating and fasting, based on what works for the body and mind the best.

The alternate-day method is like a step up from eat-stop-eat and 24-hour methods, especially if the individual truly alternates one-day fasting and the next day eating, etc. This more intense style of fasting works particularly well for people who are working on equally intense fitness regimens, surprisingly. People who are eating more calories a day than 2000 (which is true for a lot of bodybuilders and fitness buffs) will have more to gain from the alternate-day method, for you only have to cut back your eating on fasting days to about 25% of your standard caloric intake. Therefore, those fasting days can still provide solid nutritional support for fitness experts while helping them sculpt their bodies and maintain a new level of health.

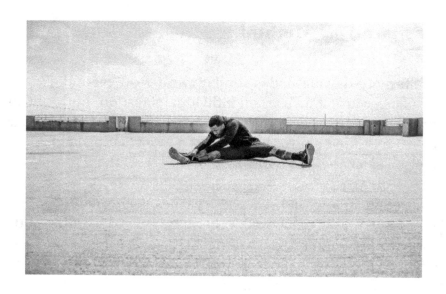

Spontaneous Skipping Method

Alternate-day method and eat-stop-eat method are certainly flexible in their approaches to when the individual fasts and when he or she eats. However, none of those mentioned above plans are quite as flexible as spontaneous skipping method. Spontaneous skipping method literally only requires that the individual skip meals within each day, whenever desired (and when it's sensed that the body can handle it).

Many people with more sensitive digestive systems or who practice more intense fitness regimens will start their experiences with IF through spontaneous skipping method before moving on to something more intensive. People who have very haphazard daily schedules or people who are around food a lot but forget to eat will benefit from this method, for it works well with chaotic schedules and unplanned energies.

Despite that chaotic and unorganized potential, spontaneous skipping method can also be more structured and organized, depending on what you make of it! For instance, someone desiring more structure can choose which meal each day they'd like to skip. Let's say he chooses to skip breakfast each day. Then, his spontaneous skipping method will be structured around making sure to skip breakfast (a.k.a.—not to eat until at least 12 pm) daily. Whatever you need to do to make this method work, try it! This method is made for experimentation and adventurousness.

Crescendo Method

The final method worth mentioning is crescendo method, which is very well-suited for female practitioners (since their anatomies can be so detrimentally sensitive to high-intensity fasts). Essentially, this approach is made for internal awareness, gentle introductions, and gradual additions, depending on what works and what doesn't. It's a very active, trial-and-error type of method.

Through crescendo method, the individual starts by only fasting 2 or 3 days a week, and on those fast days, it wouldn't be a very intense fast at all. In fact, it wouldn't even be so strict that the individual would have to consume no more than 500 calories, like with 5:2, eat-stop-eat, and others. Instead, these "fasting" days would be trial periods for methods like 12:12, 14:10, 16:8, or 20:4. The remaining 4 or 5 days out of the week would be open eating-window periods, but again, the practitioner is encouraged to maintain a healthy diet throughout the week.

Crescendo method works extremely well for female practitioners because it enables them to see how methods like 14:10 or 12:12 will affect their bodies without tying them to the method hook, line, and sinker. It allows them to see what each method does to their hormone levels, their menstruation tendencies, and their mood swings. Therefore, the crescendo method encourages these people to be more in touch with their bodies before moving too quickly into something that could do serious anatomical and hormonal damage.

Crescendo method will work extremely well for overweight or diabetic practitioners, too, for it will allow them to have these same "trial period" moments with all the methods before choosing what feels and works best, based on each individual situation.

Making Your Choice

When you make your choice from the 10 different options listed above, there are several things you'll want to keep in mind. First and foremost amongst those things will be the fact that you can always choose another method (or a more flexible one to start with) in case something doesn't work as you'd hoped. You can *always* troubleshoot your method in this way, and there's more on this topic in chapter 9 for those interested in troubleshooting (as well as for those being forced by their bodies to troubleshoot ASAP).

Ultimately, you'll also want to keep the following points in mind as you go about selecting your method: body type & abilities, lifestyle, daily tendencies, work routine, friends & family, and dietary choices. For all these considerations, remember what feels best to you, and remember to keep your goals with IF in mind at all times! If you ever feel like you're sacrificing your sanity or bodily health to attain these goals, go back to that step of troubleshooting, for you should never need to sacrifice those things to achieve any type of goals. Essentially, keep your eye on the prize and remember to choose what feels right and see what works from there.

Consider your body type and abilities. Think of how your body looks and feels and how much about it you'd like to change. Think about how you react to food and what it looks like when you're hungry. Think about those things you view as your "limits" and how comfortable you are with pushing. Are you a fitness freak or a couch potato? Are you huskier or slimmer? Does your body hold onto fat or build muscle quickly? Do you retain water weight or not? Do you work out? Do you require a lot of water when you do? Consider all these things about your body and more, then compare them to the methods listed above. Compare them, too, to your overall goals with Intermittent Fasting to make sure that you're choosing a method that will help you actualize those goals as you conceive of them. If you're looking to lose weight quickly, try a method that works with days "on" and "off" between fasting and eating. If you're looking to build muscle, lean-gains method is probably the choice for you! If you're looking to boost your brain and heart, start with crescendo method and see where it takes you!

Consider your lifestyle. When do you normally wake up and how much sleep do you get on an average night? How hungry are you normally when you do wake up? How fast is your metabolism and when do you notice its peak? How do you make your living? Do you spend a lot of time in the car or on your feet or in an office? Are you constantly around other people or are you often alone? When you choose your method for Intermittent Fasting, make sure to consider all these lifestyle points. Maybe you wouldn't want to choose to time with a method that disallows you to eat when you normally need the most energy. Maybe you wouldn't want to choose a method that forces you to eat when you're supposed to be at work. Most of these methods have a degree of choice and flexibility, so when you do find one you like, remember that you don't have to put yourself in positions that go against your nature (or circadian rhythms) to achieve any of your goals. Stay flexible, keep your goals in mind, and respect the norms of your body!

Consider your daily tendencies. Do you eat mostly in the daylight hours or after the sun goes down? Do you go to work in the daytime or nighttime? Are you generally nocturnal, diurnal, or crepuscular? Do you have a lot of freedom and flexibility in your daily routines? Do you travel a lot for work? Do you spend a lot of time on the move? Do you have trouble remembering to eat? Are you the type of person that works out on the regular? Consider these themes in your life and more before you choose your method. Does it make sense for you to have low intake days where you consume 500 calories or less? Or does it make more sense for you to have extended periods in each day where you're just not eating based on your habits or tendencies or otherwise? Plan something that makes sense and respects your habits so that the transition into Intermittent Fasting is as easy and painless as possible.

Consider your work routine. Do you go to work in the morning or night? Are you allowed to eat at work? Do you work around food or in the food service industry? Do you work on your feet all day or by doing something strenuous? Do you receive purposeful or accidental exercise opportunities at work or are you just sitting in the same position all day? All these elements of your work routine will be important to consider as you decide which avenue of Intermittent Fasting to go down. You won't want to engage in a method like 20:4 if you're at work every day for incredibly short shifts. 20:4 works better for someone who works very long and distracting days. You won't want to try a method like 12:12 if part of your eating window involves being at work, when you're not allowed to eat at work. Remember to take your work life, routines, and restrictions into account when you go about making this choice, for you will make things much less harsh on yourself if you can look at this bigger picture from the beginning and planning stages.

Consider your friends, coworkers, and family. How loud are their opinions? Are their lives oriented toward health? Do they demean you a lot or make fun of your choices? Or are they encouraging all the time? Are these people your support system or are they your devils' advocates? Do you have the sense that they want to see you succeed? On the most basic level, are they nice to you and respectful of your choices? It might not seem that important, but the attitudes and supportive capacity of your friends, coworkers, and family can mean *the world* when you make a big choice like starting Intermittent Fasting in your life. Sometimes, people just don't want to see us succeed. They block our successes with jealousy, pride, ignorance, or arrogance. When friends and family act like this, it's better to choose a method that allows you to avoid discussing IF around them whatsoever. When friends and family are open and supportive, they shouldn't influence your choice that much at all; it's just when things are tenuous that you'll need to keep them (and your time around them) in consideration.

Finally, consider your dietary choices. Do you eat a lot of processed foods? Or do you eat a largely whole-foods, plant-based diet? Do you count calories? Do you cautiously skim nutrition facts? Are you looking for something specific like high fat, high fiber, or high protein? Are you hoping to change your diet entirely or are you trying to keep things the way they are? Are you willing to sacrifice items of your diet to actualize your goals? All these questions help determine which type of method you're going to be ready for. Essentially, if you're trying to change your diet entirely, a method with days "on" and days "off" will work best for you. In this case, try 5:2, alternate-day, eat-stop-eat, and spontaneous skip methods. However, if you don't want to change your diet that much at all, a method where you fast for periods within each day will be desirable instead. Try methods like 20:4, 16:8, 14:10, or 12:12 for this type of situation.

As long as you make your selection with these 6 points in mind, you're sure to succeed with your Intermittent Fasting goals. You enable yourself to make the safest, smartest, best choice for your circumstances, and that's an incredible tool to use in so many different applications. In this case, it's a tool that will help keep you healthy, boost your brain, heal your heart, and shed that excess weight like melted butter!

As a reminder, your first choice still might not be the absolute *right one*, but by making the most educated choice possible, you're sure to start from a good place and learn a lot about yourself regardless. Make sure you have a runner-up method (or two!) that's easy to swap to just in case the first one doesn't seem to show progress. Work smarter, not harder! Plan ahead, do the research and know yourself. These are the truest steps to success that I know. And as always, don't be afraid to check with your doctor or nutritionist once the choice has been made. They'll be able to give you the final affirmation you need so you can get started on your new, healthy lifestyle with Intermittent Fasting in no time!

Chapter 7: Approaching Your Fast

It can be hard to transition into the first fasting period, but this chapter understand those struggles and comes equipped. Included in this chapter are 10 tips to getting started along with pointers on what to expect and what to look out for, and by the end, you should feel confident that your attempts at Intermittent Fasting will be productive, successful, and positive.

10 Tips to Get Started

Whether this is your first fast or your thousandth, everyone sometimes needs a little boost to get started. This section includes 10 tricks of the trade that will help you do just that.

1. Choose a method that aligns with your daily routine! When you work through chapter 6 and decide which method feels right, you don't have to choose something that's intentionally challenging. Go easy on yourself! Choose what feels like a natural extension of your daily routine. Your body, mind, and soul will thank you for it!

2. Plan your method! Don't go into your first Intermittent Fast (or yours fifth, for that matter!) without planning which method you'll choose, based on your lifestyle, routines, and tendencies.

3. Stick with your chosen method at least for the first week! You might feel tired of what you've chosen, and you might feel equally frustrated that things aren't working for you right away. But if you dedicate at *least* a week with a method, you can be sure whether or not it's helpful (and if not, you can discern how to tweak it to be better).

4. Do the research! If there's something else you've heard of (a rumor, a method, a fact, etc.) that are not included in this book, go find it! Research any questions that arise to be sure what you choose is right for *you*.

5. If you're unsure, check with your doctor or nutritionist! There are a lot of complexities involved with Intermittent Fasting, and one of the biggest complexities is the conundrum of your body. Your doctor or nutritionist will know your body and its needs best, so if you've decided on a method, run it by them to be sure that it's the one for you.

6. Alter your diet slightly ahead of time! If you're going to do a day-on, day-off style of fasting, start by cutting out snacks! Scale back what you're eating to make things easier on yourself when you start. On the other hand, if you're pairing diet with IF, start the diet *before* you start fasting so that you have a handle on that better (and so that you don't have to detox from certain foods while you're also fasting).

7. Check the nutrients you'll be receiving! Before you fast, make sure you're looking at the macronutrient levels of the foods you'll be eating. You want to make sure you have the right number of calories, carbs, proteins, and fats to stay healthy and energized.

8. Before the first day, make sure you're prepared! On the evening before your fast, make your dinner choice as conscious as possible, down to the timing. Don't gorge yourself and don't go crazy on something overly rich or decadent. Instead, eat a modest dinner that's not too late and not *too* filling. Furthermore, don't snack after dinner so that you can wake up with a decent chunk of your fast already underway.

9. Keep a lot of drinks on hand! Drinks will be pivotal for keeping your energy and spirits up, so make sure you have them and that they're

the *right* types of drinks to support IF! Check out chapter 8 for details in this respect.

10. To establish a routine, take things slow and don't be too hard on yourself! It can be hard to adjust to a whole new food-related lifestyle, so don't push yourself *too hard* too soon into the process. Stay realistic with your expectations for yourself and the fast.

What to Expect

When you start Intermittent Fasting, you'll want to keep several things in mind so that you know exactly what to expect. With these appropriate expectations in place, you'll have a much easier time troubleshooting your fast (see chapter 9) later on.

First, you'll want to <u>expect mornings to be a whole new adventure</u>. Sometimes, (based on the method you choose) your mornings will be slow and stagnant, and sometimes they'll be filled with energy. Sometimes, you may be super hungry in the morning, while other times you might be perfectly fine.

Second, expect that <u>coffee will become your new best friend</u>. Coffee will help you snap some energy when you're feeling low without food, and it can also keep you focused on something to do with your hands and mouth when you feel hungry but can't quite eat yet due to timing.

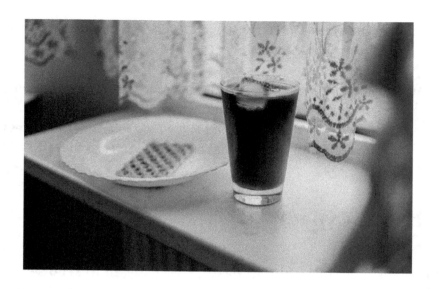

Third, expect that <u>your first week might be rough and moody</u>. You might have to build up a tolerance to all that Intermittent Fasting has to offer, but once you cross that first hurdle, you should have a much easier time moving on.

Fourth, <u>some things in your life will increase</u>. You'll become more present, more mindful, more conscious of the world and your feelings, and more conscious of how food makes you feel as well as what it makes you do and say.

Fifth, <u>some things in your life will decrease, namely your weight!</u> You could also see a decrease in sleep for the first few weeks, and while you go through the body's initial detoxification period, you might also find that your sleep isn't restful even when you can get it. Eventually, things will even out, and sleep will not be an issue anymore.

Sixth, <u>you will get cranky and emotional in the first few weeks</u>. During this period, you will be going through heavy detoxification of body and mind. You'll have to push through any anxiety, temper tantrums, and restlessness to keep your mind on the prize. You may even get a little smelly during this time as you sweat out all the bad, but your body and mind will thank you for this later!

Seventh, and finally, expect that <u>your relationship with food will completely change for the better</u>. You will be less of a slave to your cravings and desires, and you will be more understanding of people who live with less. You will be less dependent, more informed, more grateful, and less hangry when food takes a while.

While some of these expectations are relatively negative, most if not all have incredibly positive potential. Once you're through the first few weeks of your fast, you should see the silver lining of each expectation clearly.

What to Look Out For

All the above expectations should end up relatively resolved after the first week, but there will be signs in your body if things are *not* resolved and getting worse. These signs will be things to look out for, and if the situations don't improve with alteration and time, it may mean that IF isn't right for you after all. However, keep these tidbits in mind for your practice so that you can be on the lookout for your own best interest.

First, <u>watch out if you experience constant headaches, lightheadedness, or dizziness</u>. If you have these experiences just once or twice, that can be resolved, but if these arise *constantly*, there's a deeper problem that needs to be addressed.

Second, and furthermore, <u>if you're overly tired without the ability to sleep or constantly sleeping after the second week</u>, there's something wrong with your method or the way you're going about it.

Third, <u>watch out if you're getting hunger pangs that can't be dealt with</u>. Generally, during Intermittent Fasting, you'll experience hunger, and that's normal. You'll ride through the hunger wave and move past it. However, if these waves come again and again with no satiation, you might be in a bit of trouble. Check out chapter 10 for more details on this point.

Fourth, and finally, <u>watch for any severe personality changes</u>. If you start becoming obsessively compelled to practice your fast in new ways or if you feel that you're becoming overly controlling of or controlled *by* your fast, it might be time to take a break. Your personality can change, but if it does so in a way that aligns with the warnings mentioned in chapter 5, there's something to be concerned about.

These four points are all valid experiences to watch for, and if they appear without resolution, it may well be time to quit, but you can still try to troubleshoot your methods with the steps in chapter 9 before you make that call. As always, it's your body, so it's your choice. Just make sure it's the smartest and most informed choice you're capable of making.

Chapter 8: What to Eat/What Not to Eat

Before you start your first fast, however, it's helpful to know what's good to eat and drink versus what hurts the cause. This chapter is dedicated to that knowledge of what's good to eat and drink when Intermittent Fasting versus what to avoid at all costs.

10 Great Foods to Eat

When you're doing IF, you'll need to eat foods that give you enough energy to last until your next breakfast, and that can be tricky if you don't know what to look out for! This section lists 10 of the best foods to incorporate in your diet when practicing IF.

1. Avocado is high in calories and healthy fats, so it's perfect to have as a snack or in a meal.

2. Cruciferous vegetables like cauliflower, Brussel sprouts, broccoli, and more are full of fiber and so much more!

3. Potatoes of all kinds are great to satisfy one's hunger and provide a nutritional punch.

4. Legumes and beans of all varieties contain good carbohydrates that can help lower weight without too much restriction of calories.

5. Berries contain vitamin C, flavonoids, and antioxidants that will add a lot of good to your fast.

6. <u>Eggs</u> of any animal are packed with protein to help you build muscle and retain energy during the fast.

7. <u>Wild-caught fish</u> have a great amount of protein as well as vitamin D for one's brain and healthy fats and omega-3s for one's body.

8. <u>Anything high in protein</u> or <u>high in probiotic content</u> will be good to have along for the ride.

9. <u>Grains and nuts</u> are full of fiber, and healthy fats for snacks or meals during your fast's eating windows.

10. Spices such as <u>cayenne pepper, psyllium husk, or dried dandelion</u> are natural weight loss agents that can help anyone's process.

3 Foods to Avoid

On the flip side, some foods will absolutely set you back on your path to progress, and it will be equally important to know what to steer clear of. The following list includes three foods to avoid at all costs.

1. <u>Processed foods</u> will be the most important things to avoid, especially as you prepare for your fast.

2. <u>Highly GMO foods</u> are also things to avoid when you're working through your fast. They can offset the actual nutrition being provided by other foods in your diet.

3. <u>Sugary foods</u> may curb your appetite, but they won't do anything good for your body in the long run. Steer clear for your future ease.

10 Great Drinks

Even when you *are* fasting, drinks are still allowed! Make sure to choose drinks that are nutritious but not too filling, and mix it up whenever you can to keep things from getting stagnant for your taste buds (and body). 10 of the best drinks to incorporate for IF are listed below.

1. <u>Water with fruit or veggie slices</u> will provide nourishment and flavor for those times when you're fasting and need a little extra boost!

2. <u>Probiotic drinks</u> like kombucha or kefir will work to heal your gut and tide you over till the next eating window.

3. <u>Black coffee</u> will become your new best friend but be sure not to add cream and sugar! They detract from the good work coffee can do for your body during IF.

4. <u>Teas of any kind</u> are soothing as well as healing for various elements of the body, mind, and soul. Once again, be sure to omit the cream and sugar!

5. <u>Chilled or heated broths</u> made from vegetables, bone, or animals can sustain one's energy during times of fast, too.

6. <u>Apple Cider Vinegar shots</u> are great for the tummy and for healing overall! Hippocrates' remedy for any ailment included this and a healthy regimen of fasting occasionally, so you're sure to succeed with this trick.

7. <u>Water with salt</u> can provide electrolytes, hydration, and brief sustenance for anyone whose stomachs won't stop grumbling.

8. <u>Fresh-pressed juices</u> are always great for the body, mind, and soul, and in times of IF, they can sustain one's energy and mood during day-long fast periods, in particular.

9. <u>Wheatgrass shots</u> are just as healthy as ACV shots, with a whole other subset of benefits. To awaken your body and give a jolt to your system, try these on for size.

10. <u>Coconut water</u> is more hydrating than standard water, and it's full of additional nutrients, too! Try this alternative if you need some enhancement to your usual water.

3 Drinks to Avoid

On the flip side, some drinks will definitely push you back from your goals, so keep an eye out for the 3 listed below! Avoid them at all costs.

1. <u>Sodas of any kind</u>, whether diet or non-diet, are to be avoided absolutely. They are high in sugar and riddled with terrible things for your body. Try to steer clear of this drink, especially during fast periods.

2. <u>Coconut and almond drinks that are high in sugar</u> are also to be avoided. Artificial sweeteners are killers for one's blood sugar and insulin levels. They will reverse all the good work you've done, so be cautious.

3. <u>Alcohol</u> will distract you from your focus and commitment to the fast, and it will also steer your body off-course from where you want it to be. Try to IF soberly.

Chapter 9: Troubleshooting Your Fast

Sometimes, things don't go perfectly with Intermittent Fasting, but it's not hard to know what to correct when things do go down that problematic path. This chapter will lead you through troubleshooting techniques for your method, for your practice as a whole, and those sad moments when it might be time to stop. After reading this portion, you should feel safe and comforted by the knowledge that even *if* things don't work out well for you with Intermittent Fasting, there are several ways to turn things around.

5 Ways to Troubleshoot Your Method

For those times when you're not doing well, but you think the method's at fault, check in with these 5 tactics.

1. Make sure your method relies on your body's natural rhythms. If it does not, you will experience struggles and trials in your attempt to adjust to the lifestyle. To troubleshoot this issue, adjust your method of choice or change it entirely so that it lines up with your daily tendencies better.

2. If you're constantly hungry on an alternate-day method (like 5:2), troubleshoot your process by switching to a daily method (like 16:8) instead. You don't have to force yourself to fast for whole days with Intermittent Fasting! If it's not working for you, try something else like occasional eating windows each day.

3. If you're feeling gorged after your eating windows but not *full*, there are a few things you can do. Mainly, make sure you're eating

correctly each time you breakfast! You won't want to eat too quickly or too much, and these are the most common problems I've seen with IF. Eat a portion size you normally would and drink a sufficient amount of water with each meal or snack.

4. If you're getting dehydrated but still feeling okay, food- and health-wise, you might want to up the number of liquids you're taking in each day. Don't neglect liquids for the sake of focusing on food! Water, juices, teas, and more can help boost your goals, and they should never be forgotten.

5. Make sure your method of choice revolves around your work schedule, too! Especially if you work in the food industry, you'll want to plan your fasting times around periods when you know you won't be around (or tempted by) food. Spend your fasting periods in spaces that are safe, and spend this time doing things that are productive but not too strenuous. Your body and mind will thank you!

5 Ways to Pull it Back Together

On the other hand, sometimes it's not the method, it's the overall approach and strategy. In this section, you will find 5 ways to troubleshoot that avenue of the experience.

1. If you find yourself trying to force things to happen, take a step back and remember that there's only so much you can control! Your timing can only be *so* perfect, your training and exercise can only be *so* accurate, your body can only get strong *so* quickly, and your desires for otherwise are just that—desires. Don't get caught up in imposed expectations, goals, or thoughts for timing or success. Take your experience day by day and let it reveal to you what it can. The less controlling and forceful thoughts you can have, the better.

2. If you find yourself trying to stop too eagerly, say within the first week or so, remember that there's really no reason to stop (especially within the first two weeks!) unless you're experiencing one of the three signs that it's truly time to stop (listed in the section just below this one). <u>Don't give up</u>! Push through any tension and anxieties, and if your concerns linger after the end of the second week, you're likely right that IF isn't the lifestyle choice for you. However, most will find that their systems get adjusted to IF perfectly after the end of the first week and that all concerns were truly for naught.

3. <u>If you find yourself losing inspiration, try to remember what motivated you to try Intermittent Fasting in the first place</u>! Go back to chapter 3 if you need and re-read all the potential benefits! Go back to the first medical case study you read that inspired you to try IF—or talk to the person that recommended the lifestyle of IF to you. By getting back in touch with these inspirational roots, your experience will be made all the better.

4. If you find yourself getting stuck on worries or concerns for your safety, <u>remember to stay grounded in your body</u>! Don't get so excitable that you're stuck in your head, thinking the worst about things that aren't even happening to you! If you find yourself falling into these patterns of anxiety, remember to try thinking past and through these trials. On the other side, you will remember *why* you tried IF, *what good* it can do for you, and *how good* your body is already feeling because of it.

5. <u>If you find your path blocked by unappreciative or unaccepting family or friends, it might be time to get some distance from them</u>. You can reclaim your choices in life by making them purposefully in front of these people or consciously and contemplatively on your own, away from them. Based on how intense these family members' and friends' opinions are, you can choose to avoid these

people entirely, you can choose not to talk IF themes with them, or you can simply choose not to fast or breakfast around them. There are many ways to reclaim your process in instances such as this; you'll just need to remember your purpose and stand your ground (for yourself).

3 Signs it is Time to Stop

Sometimes, it's not the approach, and it's not the method either. Sometimes, it's just time to call it quits, and it's not so much about quitting as it is about saving your body. If any of the following 3 signs come up, it's probably best to stop.

1. <u>If any of your health struggles have gotten worse despite your attempts with IF, it might be time to stop</u>. Especially if you've troubleshot your plan, tried to turn it around and received no betterment to your situation, it's probably time for you to stop IF for good.

2. <u>If you experience intense burning in the pit of your stomach or pains inside your chest cavity, despite having tried to troubleshoot your method, it could be that IF is causing more problems for you than it's healing</u>. With these dangerous pains in place, stop IF and discuss these issues with your doctor or a nutritionist.

3. <u>If you vomit uncontrollably despite having eaten nothing or if you have diarrhea that's almost constant, you're not going about this right</u>. For now, just stop trying IF and discuss what's going on with your doctor or nutritionist. They will likely be able to reveal what's going wrong with your process—otherwise, it's just plain time to stop.

Chapter 10: Am I Hungry? Or Am I Starving?

One of the most confusing elements of Intermittent Fasting (especially for beginners) is how to tell when you're just hungry versus when you're in danger of starving. This chapter will lead you through several tips to control your hunger, signs of starvation, and ways to pull everything back together if starvation takes hold over hunger.

5 Tips to Control Hunger

If you can tell you're just hungry, use one of the 5 tips to counteract that belly grumble!

1. First things first, you *will* encounter hunger quite a lot. You will come to build a new relationship with hunger altogether, and you will know it as its unique feeling that's different from starvation entirely. With these feelings of hunger, it's best to <u>think of it as a wave passing through you that you can ride</u>. Once you ride the wave, it will pass and return in time, but you will teach yourself patience, stamina, and endurance by practicing this visualization for yourself.

2. If you experience occasional dizziness or lightheadedness, you're likely feeling the effects of low blood pressure or low blood volume. You can heal this lowness yourself by <u>drinking water with just a pinch of salt to restore your system's electrolytes</u>. You could also try taking magnesium supplements to correct these sensations. Remember, constant feelings of this sort are signs to stop, but occasional states like this are normal.

3. When your stomach starts to grumble literally, <u>don't be alarmed</u>! Your stomach is just working out the last bits inside it to send along to your intestinal system. These grumbles are totally natural and utterly normal. Ride through the grumbly waves just like you would for the sensation of hunger, and your stomach will stop doing its thing in just a few minutes, most likely.

4. <u>Some people experience hunger as a variety of moodiness</u>. If you tend to get "hangry" or sassy when you're hungry, there are a couple of things you can do. The most obnoxious method to deal with feelings like this is just to see if it lingers after you're fully adjusted to IF as a lifestyle. If you start feeling moody on top of being hungry, you can also choose the subtle method, which is to get introspective with yourself and try to figure out how to best these feelings for the sake of your health and growth. Essentially, if you're feeling sassy, hangry, or moody, these emotions are signs of pure hunger. They're not to be fearful of, and they're easy to troubleshoot. All you need to do is bear through it and try to be better.

5. <u>Alternate coffee and water</u> as your chosen drinks during fast periods! Yes, you're going to be hungry. Yes, you're going to want to eat. However, you're going to need to stay strong and consistently supplement foods with drinks during these fasting periods. As your right-hand-guys (drink-wise), keep coffee and water at your side constantly and make sure to alternate between the two! Just coffee will keep you hungrier more often, and just water will make you feel utterly empty without any energy. By switching between the two, you'll help your body deal with hunger in big ways.

5 Signs of Starvation

If it feels like more than just hunger, check in with these 5 signs to ensure you're not on the path to starvation.

1. The first sign of starvation mode (or the state of metabolic damage) is that your brain can't handle functions that were considered "normal" before IF. If you find your cognitive skills significantly decreased, your approach to IF is not benefitting you. You should be able to experience sharper and more purposeful cognition through the addition of IF. The opposite is absolutely a warning sign.

2. Another sign of your body going into starvation mode will be inconsistent or consistently low energy levels. For the individual experiencing the early stages of starvation, there will be intense mood and energy drops that distract from the focus and energy going into his or her day. There could also be almost constant periods of very low energy that are detrimental to the individual's day.

3. Another sign that your body might be headed in this direction would be the intense and noted loss of weight with nothing gained back in terms of muscle, despite exercise and intermittent food intake. Yes, you certainly *want to* lose weight, but there are many ways of losing weight that is healthy (in relation to IF) yet losing an excessive amount in a very short period is *not* that healthy way.

4. A couple more bodily signs of starvation mode involve excessive bloating or gas, heartburn or reflux, fluid retention in ankles, weight *gain*, loss of muscle mass, completely ceased menstruation in women, decreased immunity (or longer flu and cold periods), or severe sleep disturbances. Anyone of these signs is troubling alone, but when two or more are experienced together, you can be *sure* you're in a state of metabolic damage.

5. A few final mental and emotional signs of starvation mode include severe mood swings, a prevalence of depression or anxiety

(especially where there was none before IF), lowered libido, seriously lowered energy, or lack of interest in living. Any of these signs alone is detrimental enough to warrant concern, so if any of these experiences arise for you, it may be time to stop IF for good.

3 More Ways to Pull it Back Together

Once you're able to tell the level of threat you're at (if it's hunger or truly starvation), there are other ways to pull things back together and get the practice going once more. 3 of those approaches are listed below.

1. If you've troubleshoot your hunger, and you're ready to go back for more, think harder about what snacks and meals you're eating when you breakfast! You can eat highly-nourishing, calorie-dense foods that have healthy fats and all the proteins your body could need. Don't neglect your responsibilities along with that ability! It's up to *you* to choose the healthy options and to purposefully feed yourself with living, healing foods.

2. For those who get too close to (or too deep into) starvation mode, you can bring things back together by taking a few days off of the fast entirely. Take a break and come back to things with a refreshed mind and reinvented plan of attack. With a new method and mental approach—as well as the unfortunate experience of starvation— your IF adventure can be completely re-engaged for the better.

3. If you've struggled with hunger and starvation, you might be able to practice your version of IF that isn't listed in chapter 6 in this book at all. Based on your body and your experience, you may be able to completely invent your own, holistic approach to IF that no one else has ever thought of before. Perhaps your approach needs certain timing in each day to work. Perhaps it requires certain foods and

not others. Perhaps it requires the support of others and a specific setting. Perhaps it needs the right mindfulness to not lead to starvation. Whatever they happen to be, with your failures under your belt, you will learn what works for you and what doesn't, which gives you the unique opportunity to invent your Intermittent Fast from scratch to incorporate the complexities of your experience. Embrace that potential and try again if you're able!

Chapter 11: Flavors of Fasting

Intermittent Fasting is great for the body, mind, and soul for a variety of reasons. This chapter shows the many different applications of Intermittent Fasting. For example, it can be productive for weight loss, heart health, brain health, depression, and so much more, and this chapter will give you those inside scoops.

Fasting for Weight Loss

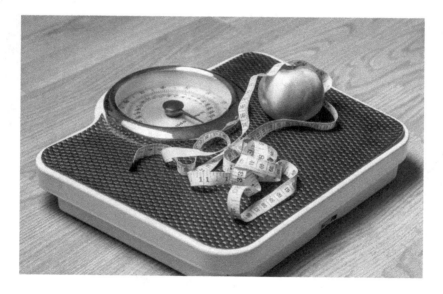

For the body, Intermittent Fasting works magic with weight loss. By eating less, eating less often, or eating more consciously, practitioners restrict their intake of calories, which is almost guaranteed to have weight loss effects in the body. For the practitioner fasting 15 hours a day, there's a trajected loss of about 3 pounds of fat each week. That's without any attempt at dieting or exercise. When it comes down to it, Intermittent

Fasting is positively correlated with weight loss 100% of the time. Give it a try to get rid of that pesky belly fat! You'll be so glad you did—as long as you're up to the commitment!

Fasting for Diabetes

For the body and mind, Intermittent Fasting is helpful about those with Types 1 or 2 diabetes. A low-intensity approach to IF will enable the individual with diabetes to experience more consistent energy levels, more glucose absorption into the cells, and more weight loss that's productive than ever before. To be clear, IF is not a cure for diabetes, and it does still pose some issues, but as long as the practice is low-intensity and taken with care, the individual is sure to see significant growth of both body and mind.

Fasting for Heart Health

Just like with diabetes, Intermittent Fasting doesn't cure heart disease, but it can definitely make things better! In specific, relating to heart health, IF can enable the body to have lower blood pressure, lower cholesterol levels, less triglycerides, and fewer instances of inflammation. All of which contribute to heart disease (and worse). Anyone dealing with heart struggles is invited to try IF, for it can reverse potentially disastrous circumstances with just a few lifestyle changes.

Fasting for Brain Health

Intermittent Fasting can do incredible things for one's brain. It's crazy to think that people dealing with mental struggles of dementia, Alzheimer's, and more can have their situations eased with consistent periods of low caloric intake! It's even crazier once you know *how* IF helps these individuals. In specific, IF can cause the literal growth of new brain cells, and it can make one's cognition heightened even in times of distress. It can increase neuroplasticity overall, and it can help the brain & body learn how to burn fat for fuel in addition to just sugar (which is the main issue for people with diabetes!). Fat burns cleaner and more efficiently as fuel for the body and brain. Finally, IF can also give a gigantic boost to one's energy levels, which easily relates to one's brain power. Try Intermittent Fasting for your body, and you'll be elated to see what also can happen in your brain!

Fasting in Medicine

Fasting has been used for medical reasons for decades, too, and those medical reasons are extremely varied! Even today, before a routine surgery, your surgeon will tell you not to eat or drink anything past a certain hour. Before a serious check-up requiring intensive procedures, your doctor might ask you to do the same. Even before our pets go to get surgeries, their veterinarians will ask we not feed them past a certain time. Then there are the words of Hippocrates and Paracelsus (among others) from ancient Greece, both of whom advocated for fasting to enact medical health. From ages across time to today, fasting has been used to further medical procedures and to encourage overall healing for patients with a variety of conditions.

Fasting for Cancer

There are so many benefits of Intermittent Fasting, but none are so profound as its abilities to aid cancer patients. Recent studies have proven that IF both decreases cancer regrowth rates, as well as the risk of cancer in individual practitioners. These effects are most often related to IF's abilities to lower glucose production, to boost the creation of tumor-killing cells, to rebuild the immune system and each cell at a time, and to balance one's nutritional consumption. Altogether, these effects work wonders for people battling life's most terrifying disease.

Fasting for Depression

While Intermittent Fasting can have such healing effects on body, mind, and soul that cancer symptoms are lessened in intensity or erased in entirety, it also has the same three-fold effects for individuals battling depression. The World Health Organization has stated that depression is on the rise across the globe, yet its symptoms and effects on the body, mind, and soul are so various that it's hard to tackle any one element at a time. Thankfully, Intermittent Fasting addresses many elements at once, healing all of them in kind. IF's effects on hormone production throughout the body have sensational consequences that align with increased mood, lessened anxiety, and a greater sense of well-being and purpose.

Chapter 12: Q & A

To wrap things up before our final chapter of recipes, this section is all about those final questions that might linger in your mind. It's about addressing your concerns and putting your mind at ease. If you have a question that doesn't appear to be answered anywhere in this book, ask to your trusted nutritionist and make sure to do things right.

15 Questions & Answers about IF

Whether they're about methods, strategies, approaches, measurements of success, or otherwise, these questions (and their respective answers) should address any lingering concerns or confusions for any future (or current) IF practitioners.

1. Who is Intermittent Fasting for?

   IF is actually for anyone! It works best for people who are simply serious about making their health better and about changing their weights for the better without sacrificing their diets.

2. What should I consider before my first fast?

   Think of your bodily limitations, your daily routine, your work schedule, and your tendencies with hunger and thirst. The more you know about yourself, the better! On the other hand, the more you know about the method you're going to try, the better, too! Consider every detail you can, from your personality to your body weight, your tendencies, your cravings, and more. Together, all these details will help you make your first fast the best and most lasting change in your life.

3. If I'm diabetic, should I try IF?

Absolutely! Give IF a try, but don't be too strict with diet or exercise while you attempt it. Additionally, don't be too strict with your timing or snack restriction. Diabetic individuals can experience troubles with IF when they limit themselves too much, so make sure you're not sacrificing your health but definitely give it a try!

4. Will IF help with more than weight loss?

Yes, definitely! Intermittent Fasting can heal the brain, the heart, the digestive system, the mood, and so much more! It's not just about weight loss, and anyone who insists it is just lying to you.

5. Which method of IF is best?

The answer to this question is more subjective than objective. There's no one method that's best for everyone. In fact, each individual should choose the method that works best for him or her based on the guidelines listed in chapter 6.

6. Where should I begin if I'm interested in IF?

Start by doing some reading! Research IF and see what it can do for you. Then, start making the simple steps to your own IF transition. These simple steps include snacking less, eating less often late at night, waiting a little longer to eat in the morning, and making sure to eat dinner a little bit earlier.

7. I'm breastfeeding—should I try IF or wait until I'm done?

Great question! Generally, I suggest you waiting until you're done breastfeeding to try IF or to reinstate it again. While you're breastfeeding, your body needs a specific subset of nutrients to produce what your baby needs. With an intense exercise regimen and practice of caloric restriction, you may do more harm to your body and your baby than good. It's not worth the risk, but as I wrote above, there's a possibility. For more details, check my other book *Intermittent Fasting for Women: Learn How You Can Use This Science to Support Your Hormones, Lose Weight, Enjoy Your Food, and Live a Healthy Life Without Suffering from Your Dietary Habits*

8. Should I exercise while I try IF?

As you transition into IF, start by trying to exercise occasionally, but don't expect that you'll be able to exercise as much as you had been without IF. Start small and build up to see what your body can handle, given the restricted intake. Women and diabetic individuals are almost exclusively recommended to *not* exercise while attempting IF. The consequences are too problematic for me to want you to push those boundaries.

9. Should I diet while I try IF?

You can certainly try! However, most people will realize that strict dieting does *not* pair all that well with IF unless it's the Keto Diet. People who diet by calorie counting will *not* benefit by taking this strategy into IF. People who diet by restricting protein or fat will equally *not* benefit with IF. Therefore, if you *do* combine dieting and IF, make sure your diet isn't too strict, and leave wiggle room for growth and troubleshooting. If you're attempting the Keto Diet, with its helpful divisions of fat, protein, and carbs, you may find that your diet is perfect for IF. As always, take things one day at a time, and don't cling too harshly to your diet! There may be times when it helps, but there will be times when it doesn't. Just stay open to changes and fluctuations in your experience.

10. I'm working on IF right now—why do I have a headache constantly?

Not everyone feels this type of head pain while fasting, but it is more often women than men that go through this experience. Due to studies done on Islamic peoples observing Ramadan, we can tell that the cause to this pain is not always dehydration. In fact, it's much more related to the kind of headache one gets after quitting coffee drinking. Essentially, it's a withdrawal symptom from something, and it *will* fade and go away after you keep practicing the fast. If it doesn't go away, it might be time to stop (see chapter 9).

11. Is it okay to drink during IF or is it strictly no intake?

It's absolutely acceptable (and even recommended!) for individuals to drink during fast periods. Just try to make sure your drink has no calories (so no soda, not a lot of juice, etc.), and you should be aligned with your goals! Simply remember that fasting periods are supposed to be times of rest for your body and mind, so you won't want to add anything too intense to that bodily mix in these moments. Keep the calories of the drink low, and you'll be set.

12. If I take supplements and vitamins each day, should I stop them while trying IF?

The short answer to this question is yes. The longer answer to this question is that you might want to hold off on taking your supplements on days when you're fully fasting. However, if you're not doing day-on, day-off fasts but fasting and eating within each day instead, you should have no problem continuing to take all supplements daily, as you normally would.

13. Will IF screw up my metabolism?

Your metabolism is much more connected to your body fat than most people know and are taught. Therefore, all concerns over messing up one's metabolism through IF are largely unfounded. The truth is that as your body fat goes down, so will your metabolism. The less you have to burn, the less intensely your metabolism works, but that's all balanced out by the body's natural processes. Essentially, there's no way you can screw this up.

14. Is IF safe for pregnant women and expecting mothers?

Many different groups hotly debates this, but the gist of the answer is that it depends on the mother, the situation, and the advice of the mother's doctor. Sometimes, IF poses no threat, while other times it's disastrous. Err on the side of caution and speak with your doctor or nutritionist first.

15. I have hypothyroid. Should I try IF or not?

With hypothyroid, you should still be able to try IF! The trick for you will be to make sure you never fast for more than a day at a time. Your bodily rhythms will be greatly distressed if you attempt to fast more than 24 hours at once.

Chapter 13: 15 Recipes for IF on the Keto Diet

For this recipe portion, I've mixed the Keto Diet in with our attempts for Intermittent Fasting because the two pairs so easily. Typically, the Keto Diet is divided into the following nutritional percentages: around 70% of calories from fat, around 20% of calories from protein (a moderate amount), and no more than 10% of calories from carbohydrates.

The main focus of the Keto Diet is to remove excess carbohydrates from one's diet to enable the increased production of ketones in the body, which are essentially molecules that produce fuel for the individual. With less glucose, or blood sugar, in the body (resulting from that restriction of carbohydrates), the liver breaks down fat cells and produces ketones instead. Therefore, the body runs mostly off fat and burns fat more consistently because fat becomes *essential* for its ability to breakdown into ketones (a.k.a.—energy for brain and body).

With this increased production of ketones, the body becomes slimmer and fit, less bulked with fat, less sugar-crazed, and more energized even if the individual is intermittently fasting as well. In fact, Intermittent Fasting increases the body's production of ketones differently (by producing ketosis, a fruitful metabolic state), so the two pair well together in that ketonic connection.

As a general warning, just like with Intermittent Fasting, some body types will not do well with this type of metabolic shift. If you are diabetic, breastfeeding, or taking medication for high blood pressure and you still want to attempt Intermittent Fasting, I do not recommend adding the Keto Diet to the mix. For the rest of my readers, this section should help to solidify those weight loss and lifestyle goals in no time.

Breakfasts

Low-carb breakfasts might seem counter-intuitive, but they're not only just possible! They're also delicious, nutritious, and packed with productive energy. Whichever of the two recipes below you choose, your mornings are sure to give you exactly the boost you need, and if you need more options, there are surely other sources at your disposal.

Frittata with Spinach and Mushrooms

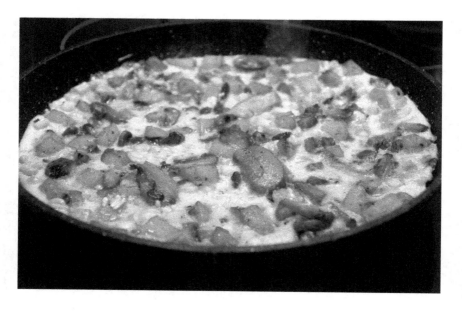

Tasty, simple, and packed with nutrition, this breakfast is best for sharing with a group of people (so there are no leftovers!) to get your day started.

This recipe needs 10 minutes of prep and about 35 minutes of cooking. It will make 4 helpings.

- Fat—59 g
- Protein—27 g
- Net Carbs—4.1 g
- Calories—661

What to Use:

- Butter (2 tablespoons)
- Bacon (6 ounces, coarsely diced)
- Spinach (8 ounces)
- Eggs (8, large-sized)
- Heavy Cream (1 cup)
- Shredded Cheese (6 ounces)
- Salt & Pepper (to taste)

What to Do:

- Start by heating the oven to 350 degrees while bringing the 2 tablespoons of butter to medium heat in a frying pan on the stovetop.
- When heated, add bacon to pan and cook until desired crispiness. Then add the spinach and stir together until soft. Remove both from pan and drain the fat. Set to the side for now.
- In a separate medium-sized bowl, combine the eggs and cream. Once whisked together, grease a 9x9 baking dish and pour the mixture in.
- Stir in bacon, spinach, and any shredded cheese. Put dish and mixture in the oven.
- Bake 30 minutes until perfectly browned.

Pancakes with Berries

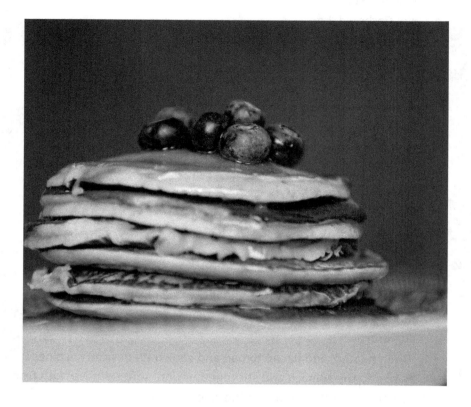

"How do you make low-carb pancakes?!" you might be asking yourself, and the answer is just within reach! These pancakes have a unique flavor, but they're nutritionally amazing and great for starting your day.

This recipe needs 5-10 minutes of prep and about 20 minutes of cooking. It will make 4 helpings.

- Fat—39 g
- Protein—13 g
- Net Carbs—5 g
- Calories—425

What to Use:

- Eggs (4, large-sized)
- Cottage Cheese (7 ounces)
- Psyllium Husk Powder (1 tablespoon)
- Butter or Coconut Oil (2 ounces)
- Berries (0.5 cup, for topping)

What to Do:

- In a medium-sized mixing bowl, stir together the first three ingredients and let sit. After about 10 minutes, the mixture should be perfectly thickened.
- Grab a large-sized non-stick skillet and heat butter or coconut oil until melted. Portion out 0.5-cup scoops of the batter onto the skillet and cook 4 minutes on each side until done.
- Prepare berries as desired (sliced or whole, etc.), and top finished pancakes with them for a delightful boost of sweetness.

Lunch

For lunch, let's not do something too big or too packed with sugar. Salads, half-wraps, stir-fries, and chicken salads will do just fine! Regardless of your tastes, there should be something to suit your pallet in this section. Given your goals and vision for Intermittent Fasting, you're bound to see progress with these recipes in no time.

Pulled Pork Sliders

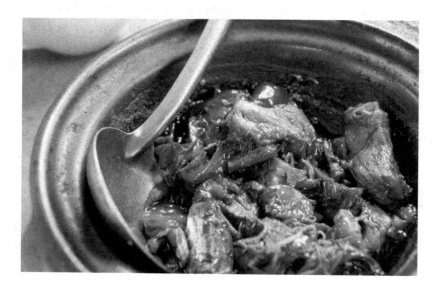

With its homemade sauce and perfect tenderness, this slider will make you feel gleeful and packed with energy to keep your intermittent fast going strong for the rest of the day.

This recipe needs 20 minutes of prep and about 45 minutes of cooking. It will make 4 helpings.

- Fat—15.1 g

- Protein—9.1 g
- Net Carbs—3.6 g
- Calories—184

What to Use:

- Pork Roast (3 pounds, boneless, cut into inch pieces)
- Butter (1 tablespoon)
- Salt (2 teaspoons)
- Garlic Powder (2 teaspoons)
- Onion Powder (1 teaspoon)
- Black Pepper (1 teaspoon)
- Smoked Paprika (1 tablespoon)
- Tomato Paste (2 tablespoons)
- Apple Cider Vinegar (0.5 cup)
- Coconut Aminos (2 tablespoons)
- Bone Broth (0.5 cup)
- Butter (0.25 cup, melted)

What to Do:

- Trim any fat from your pork roast and then cut it into appropriate chunks.
- In a small-sized bowl, combine salt, paprika, pepper, onion and garlic powders and then rub the mixture onto the pork.
- Grab a large-sized skillet and melt the tablespoon of butter before adding your chunks of pork to the skillet as well.
- In a separate, medium-sized bowl, combine all other ingredients and pour over the pork in the skillet.
- Boil the mixture to start then simmer for 30 minutes until meat is tender and is easy to pull apart in the sauce.
- Serve on low-carb bread alternative or eat in portions alone.

Curry Chicken Half-Wraps

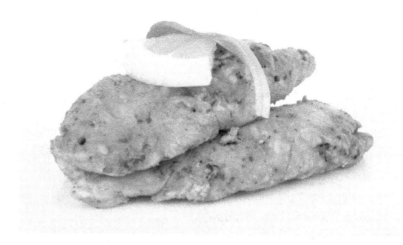

With a little effort, these half-wraps can be substituted for lettuce wraps, but they're just as delicious either way! Have as many as you need to keep that energy up throughout your day. There is a little less fat in this recipe than there could be, but you can correct that (as you like) by adding a little more cream as your garnish, or you could add a sprinkle of feta cheese on top, too. ·

This recipe needs 5 minutes of prep and about 20 minutes of cooking. It will make 2 helpings.

- Fat—36.4 g
- Protein—50.9 g
- Net Carbs—7.2 g
- Calories—554

What to Use:

- Chicken Thighs (1 pound, boneless & skinless)
- Onion (0.25 cup, minced)
- Garlic (2 cloves, minced)

- Curry Powder (2 teaspoons)
- Salt (1.5 teaspoons)
- Butter (3 tablespoons)
- Cauliflower Rice (1 cup)
- Low-Carb Wraps (cut into halves)
  - Or lettuce leaves
- Yogurt or Sour Cream (0.25 cup, for garnish)

What to Do:

- Start by preparing your chicken thighs; cut them into one-inch pieces.
- Take a large-sized skillet and heat 2 of the 3 tablespoons of butter on the skillet at medium heat. Add onion and cook till soft and browned.
- Stir in chicken pieces, garlic, and salt. Cook for about 10 minutes.
- Stir in the last tablespoon of butter, curry powder, and cauliflower rice. Cook about 5 minutes longer.
- Serve in lettuce leaves or half-wraps, and top with a scoop of cream! Enjoy.

Sautéed Mushrooms & Bacon with Greens

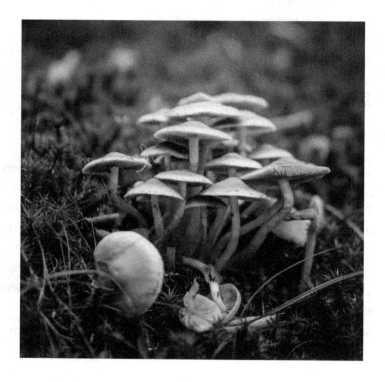

With a modest side-salad, this entrée is both elegant and appropriately filling. You'll want to bring it out when friends come around—or even for date night! The possibilities are endless.

This recipe needs 10 minutes of prep and about 10 minutes of cooking. It will make 2 helpings.

- Fat—14 g
- Protein—15 g
- Net Carbs—8.4 g
- Calories—257

What to Use:

- Bacon (4 slices, cut into half-inch pieces)
- Mushrooms (2 cups, halved; your choice)
- Salt (0.5 teaspoon)
- Thyme (2 sprigs fresh herb, destemmed)
- Garlic (3 cloves, minced)
- Greens (2 cups; your choice)
- Salad Dressing (0.25 cup; your choice)

What to Do:

- Assemble the side-salad quickly by taking your choice of greens and sprinkling on a bit of dressing. Set aside or place in the refrigerator for just a few moments.
- Take a large-sized skillet and bring to medium heat. Add bacon and cook until desired crispiness is reached. Stir in mushrooms and bring to browned color.
- Stir in salt, thyme leaves, and garlic. Cook 5 minutes then serve hot alongside your salad.

Easy Chicken Salad

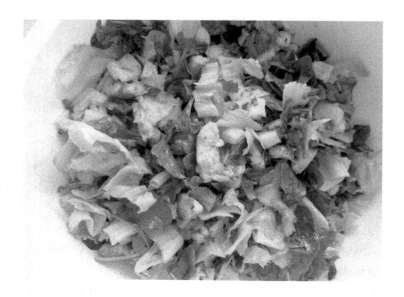

With a bread substitute of your choosing or over greens, this chicken salad will do just the trick. It even adds an interesting flavor spin on the traditional chicken salad that you can either appreciate or alter to your preferences. There is a little less fat in this recipe than what is typical of the Keto Diet, and you can correct that (for your liking) by adding more mayo or a bit of cheese to your salad as well.

This recipe needs 1 hour and 30 minutes of prep and about 15 minutes of cooking. It will make 6 helpings.

- Fat—19 g
- Protein—24.8 g
- Net Carbs—1.1 g
- Calories—279

What to Use:

- Chicken Breast (1.5 pound)

- Celery (3 stalks, sliced)
- Mayo (0.5 cup)
- Brown Mustard (2 teaspoons)
- Salt (0.5 teaspoon)
- Dill (2 tablespoons, fresh & chopped)
- Pecans (0.25 cup, chopped)

What to Do:

- Heat the oven to 425 degrees and line a baking sheet with parchment paper, aluminum foil, or baking spray.
- Add chicken breast and cook until done throughout. This will take about 15 minutes.
- Cool the breast completely. This can take anywhere from 10-30 minutes. Once cooled, cut into bite-size pieces.
- Take a large-sized bowl and stir everything except the dill and pecans together.
- Cover and chill about 1 hour before adding in dill and pecans. Serve cold.

Dinner

For dinner tonight, let's try something simple. No need for a bunch of different devices or kitchen appliances. No need for fancy spices and hours upon hours of prep. These dinner recipes are easy and accessible, yet they don't sacrifice any bit of flavor potential. They're bound to give your taste buds a delight while providing all the energy you need and fill you up for your next stint of fasting.

Single-Pan Fajita Steak

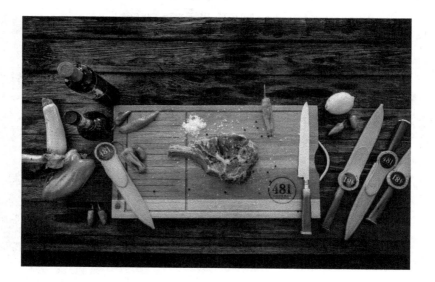

With just one sheet pan, this recipe comes together quickly and packs quite the punch for flavor! Combine it with low-carb tortillas of your choosing, eat over greens, or munch as-is. This dish is sure to please.

This recipe needs 5 minutes of prep and about 15 minutes of cooking. It will make 5 helpings.

- Fat—33 g
- Protein—31 g
- Net Carbs—5 g
- Calories—440

What to Use:

- Garlic (2 cloves, minced)
- Onion (1 medium-sized, sliced thinly)
- Chili Powder (1 teaspoon)
- Cumin (1 tablespoon)
- Salt & Pepper (to taste)
- Coconut Oil (0.25 cup)
- Lime (1, juiced & zested)
- Lemon (1, juiced & zested)
- Steak (1 pound, sliced into strips)
- Red Pepper (1 large-sized, sliced into strips)
- Yellow Pepper (1 large-sized, sliced into strips)

What to Do:

- Prepare the meat and vegetables and then stir all ingredients together on a lined or greased baking sheet.
- Preheat oven to 350 degrees then bake for 15 minutes. Half-way through the process, stir the mixture well.
- Serve with an extra sprinkle of lime juice.

Salmon Seared with Light Cream Sauce

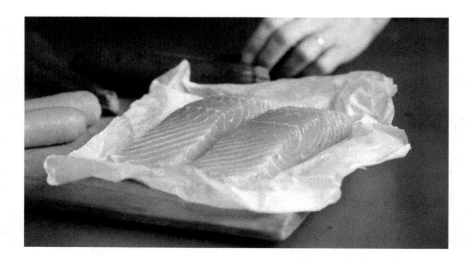

With just a handful of ingredients and a few simple steps, this recipe is gloriously easy and even more delicious than you could ever imagine. Trust me. Try it.

This recipe needs 5 minutes of prep and about 25 minutes of cooking. It will make 6 helpings.

- Fat—30 g
- Protein—54 g
- Net Carbs—2 g
- Calories—494

What to Use:

- Olive Oil (2 tablespoons)
- Salmon Fillets (3, 6-ounce fillets)
- Garlic (2 cloves, minced)
- Light Cream (1 cup)
- Cream Cheese (1 ounce)
- Capers (2 tablespoons)

- Lemon Juice (1 tablespoon)
- Dill (2 teaspoons, fresh OR 1 tablespoon, dried)
- Parmesan Cheese (2 tablespoons, grated)

What to Do:

- Grab a medium-sized skillet and heat the oil to start. Add the salmon fillets once heated through and cook 5 minutes on each side.
- Set fish aside to get the sauce together.
- In that same pan, add garlic and cook on medium heat for 2 minutes. Add cream, cream cheese, lemon juice, and capers. Simmer for 5 minutes or until thickened.
- Once thickening begins, return salmon to pan and spoon the sauce over each of the fillets.
- On low heat now, bring the salmon to the appropriate temperature. Garnish with dill and parmesan and serve!

Parmesan Bacon-Asparagus Roll-Ups

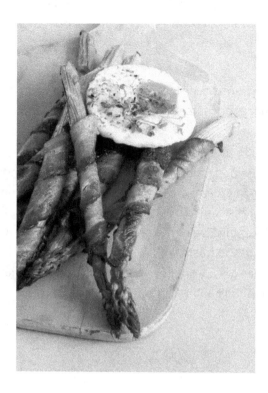

With the perfect touches of sweetness from the maple-flavored syrup and char from the baking process, these roll-ups are either the best treat ever or the perfect small meal. Enjoy as many as you like. If you need more protein than is provided in this recipe, an easy fix would be to make a chicken breast on the side. The flavor boost would be incredible with that addition, too!

This recipe needs 15 minutes of prep and about 40 minutes of cooking. It will make 2 helpings.

- Fat—23 g
- Protein—7 g
- Net Carbs—10.8 g

- Calories—257

What to Use:

- Maple-Flavored Syrup (0.5 cup)
- Butter (0.5 cup)
- Salt (0.5 teaspoon)
- Black Pepper (0.25 teaspoon)
- Asparagus (2 pounds, washed & ends removed)
- Bacon (8 slices, thick bacon)
- Parmesan (2 tablespoons + 2 teaspoons, grated)

What to Do:

- Start by preheating oven to 425 degrees.
- Then, grab a small-sized pot and bring it to medium-low heat on the stove top. Add syrup, butter, salt, and pepper. Whisk together until smooth and heated through. Set aside for later.
- Divide your 2 pounds of asparagus into 8 equal-sized groups. Wrap each group with a strip of bacon and secure the ends with toothpicks, as needed.
- Line greased baking sheet with asparagus/bacon bundles then pour over with syrup mixture and half the parmesan.
- Bake in the oven for 30 minutes. Then, switch to broil and bring the rack to the top shelf of the oven.
- Broil 2 minutes until crispy and partially-charred.
- Serve with toothpicks removed and enjoy!

Unforgettable Spaghetti Squash

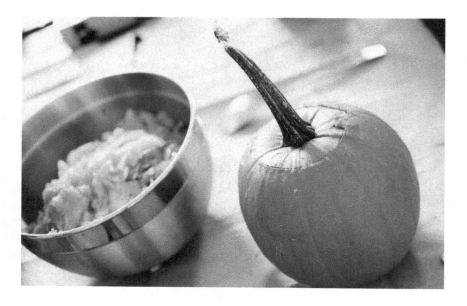

If you're like me and somewhat picky with winter squash, you're bound to be as amazed as I was when you try this spaghetti squash recipe. No pasta required, given the unique nature of this squash, and with the cheese and garlic topping, even picky eaters will surprise themselves by how much they like it. There's a little less protein in this meal than there could be, but you can boost your version by adding a little meat (try chorizo or bacon!) into the mix or by compensating through another snack or meal in the day instead.

This recipe needs 10 minutes of prep and about 1 hour of cooking. It will make 4 helpings.

- Fat—24.4 g
- Protein—8 g
- Net Carbs—3.1 g
- Calories—274

What to Use:

- Spaghetti Squash (1 medium-sized OR equivalent of 3 pounds)
- Garlic (3 cloves, minced)
- Olive Oil (1 teaspoon)
- Spinach (half-pound, chopped)
- Heavy Cream (0.5 cup)
- Parmesan Cheese (0.5 cup)
- Salt & Pepper (to taste)
- Mozzarella (grated for topping)

What to Do:

- First, preheat the oven to 400 degrees.
- Prepare the spaghetti squash by cutting it in half (lengthwise) and pulling out any seeds.
- Line a baking sheet or grease it and lay spaghetti squash with the cut side down on the sheet. Roast 30-40 minutes until easily stabbed through with a fork.
- Meanwhile, prepare the sauce. In a medium-sized pot, heat olive oil and garlic for no more than 5 minutes. Stir in spinach, cream, and parmesan in turn.
- Season with salt and pepper and set aside.
- When squash has finished roasting, pull it out from oven and begin to pull apart the strands of the squash itself (its name should make sense to you now if it didn't already!).
- With the squash threads freed, pour the cheese mixture onto the squash and into the inner "boat" part. Top with extra parmesan and mozzarella, as desired, then bake at 350 degrees for 20 additional minutes.
- At the last second, switch oven to broil and bring cheese to a beautiful browned color. Enjoy hot!

Snacks

When it comes to snacking as an Intermittent Faster, these food breaks are no joke. They're essential and important in more ways than you know. If you've chosen an IF method that relies on periodic snacks, even if you're feeling good when approaching snack time, I encourage you to *never skip those snacks*. The two listed below are packed with nutritional potential, and they're beyond easy to make. If nothing else, at least keep these two on hand, and things should be consistently productive in your IF adventure.

Hard-Boiled Eggs

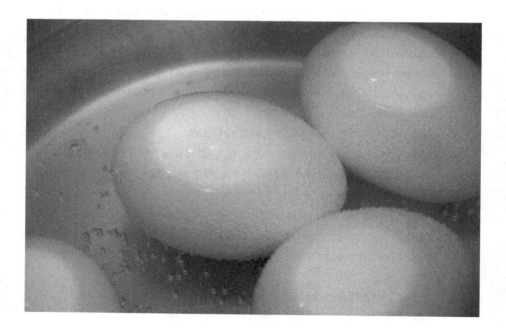

The most basic and reliable snack of all time is possibly the hard-boiled egg. With the right sprinkle of salt and pepper on top, it's hard to go wrong.

This recipe needs 5-10 minutes of cooking. It will make 4 helpings.

- Fat—29 g
- Protein—11 g
- Net Carbs—1 g
- Calories—316

What to Use:

- Eggs (8, large-sized)
- Salt & Pepper (to taste)

What to Do:

- Take a small-sized pot and fill it ¾ of the way with water. Bring to boil.
- Carefully, lay the eggs into the water and boil anywhere from 5-10 minutes. 5 minutes makes a softer egg, while 10 makes a firm and hard-boiled egg.
- Serve with topping of salt & pepper or otherwise.

Perfect Keto & IF Guacamole

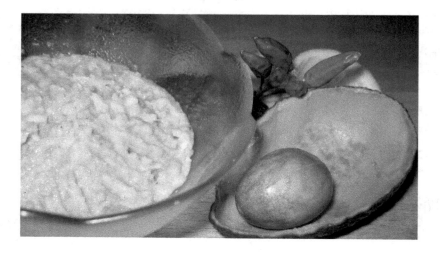

Add or subtract ingredients at will here to get your desired flavor. Going wrong with guacamole is hard! I like to add a dash of hot sauce to mine. Can't wait to see what you try. There is a little less protein than desired for proper Keto proportioning in this recipe, but you can fix that ratio with your choice of dippers or through your meal options later or earlier in the day.

This recipe needs 5-10 minutes of prep only. It will make 2 helpings.

- Fat—15 g
- Protein—3 g
- Net Carbs—13 g
- Calories—180

What to Use:

- Avocados (2 ripe ones, mashed)
- Garlic Powder (1 tablespoon)
- Onion Powder (0.5 tablespoon)

- Lime Juice (2 teaspoons)
- Salt (to taste)
- Cilantro (2 tablespoons, diced finely)
- Chili Powder or Hot Sauce (to taste)

What to Do:

- Once the avocado is mashed, stir in the garlic and onion powders along with any chili powder or hot sauce.
- As a final step, stir in lime juice and cilantro then salt to taste.
- Serve with chips or vegetable dippers!

Desserts

Dessert! The naughty word of any diet has been reclaimed in the IF / Keto Diet, for you don't always have to sacrifice treats when you're working to lose weight. The trick is to lose the carbs, stock up on fats, and add a sprinkle of protein instead. Your body will always thank you for these types of desserts, for they're designed for you to flourish (and still lose that weight!) absolutely.

No-Bake Pistachio Dessert Rounds

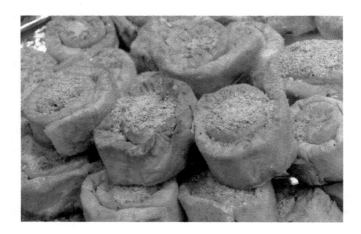

This sweet treat is easy to turn into a savory snack by just swapping out the vanilla and sweetener for garlic and fresh herbs, but it's a tasty mouth-popper either way. For dessert, this creamy and crunchy delight is sure to satisfy. As with most desserts, you lose a little by way of protein in favor of carbohydrates for this recipe, but you can make up for that with your other meals for the day, based on the method you're using.

This recipe needs 5-10 minutes of prep only. It will make 4 helpings.

- Fat—12 g
- Protein—1 g
- Net Carbs—0.5 g
- Calories—121

What to Use:

- Mascarpone Cheese (1 cup, softened)
- Vanilla Extract (0.25 teaspoon)
- Confectioner's Style Erythritol Sweetener (3 tablespoons)
- Pistachios (0.25 cup, chopped finely)

What to Do:

- In a small-sized bowl, stir together the cheese, vanilla, and sweetener. Make smooth and well-combined.
- Roll into balls. There should be about 10 1-inch diameter balls.
- Take the pistachios and chop them finely. Put onto a plate and roll the cheese balls in that pistachio powder.
- Set in refrigerator 30 minutes or more before eating. With right refrigeration, these will keep for up to one week. They will keep in the freezer for 3 months.

No-Bake Chocolate-Topped Coconut Cookies

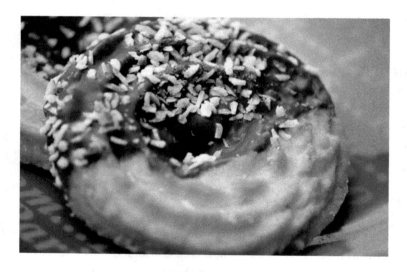

With a simple lattice of chocolate icing to top things off, these cookies are pretty to look at and even more delicious to munch on. Try and stop yourself from going back for seconds. There is a little less protein than desired for perfect Keto proportioning in this recipe, but you can balance that out by choosing a savory meal that boosts your protein and loses the carbs instead.

This recipe needs 5-10 minutes of prep. It will make 4 helpings.

- Fat—34.2 g
- Protein—3 g
- Net Carbs—8.6 g
- Calories—150

What to Use:

- Shredded Coconut (3 cups, ensure UNsweetened)
- Coconut Oil (just under 0.5 cup)
- Xylitol (0.5 cup)
- Vanilla (2 teaspoons)

- Salt (just under 0.5 teaspoon)
- Chocolate / Carob Chips (melted for drizzle)

What to Do:

- Put all ingredients except the chocolate into a blender. Process by pulsing until everything sticks together. Don't go so smooth as to make a liquid "butter" mixture.
- Once desired consistency is achieved, pour out and roll into 1-inch diameter balls. Refrigerate as desired while melting chocolate.
- Drizzle with melted chocolate in lines or a lattice. Serve chilled.

High-Protein Moussed-Up Jell-O

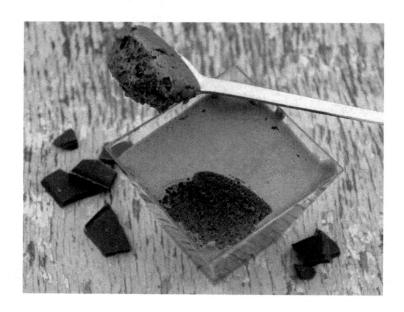

Although this recipe favors a cherry-flavored Jell-O, you can feel free to try any flavor you like! The picture above suggests chocolate, but honestly, the sky's the limit, and the outcome is just as wonderful no matter what flavor base you choose. Be sure to report back on any creative favorites!

This recipe needs 5-10 minutes of prep only. It will make 4 helpings.

- Fat—25 g
- Protein—20 g
- Net Carbs—3 g
- Calories—97

What to Use:

- Black Cherry Jell-O (1 small box, sugar-free)
- Water (0.5 cup)

- Greek Yogurt (10 ounces, plain flavored)
- Whey Protein Powder (2 scoops, unflavored)

What to Do:

- In a small-sized pot, bring water to warm yet not boiling temperature.
- Take a medium-sized mixing bowl and stir together Jell-O mix and water. Now, pour everything else into the mixing bowl and combine until perfectly smooth.
- Pour into portion bowls, ramekins, or one large bowl and refrigerate until firm, according to the Jell-O box's instructions.
- Enjoy chilled!

Conclusion

Thank you so much for making it to the end of *Intermittent Fasting*! I'm excited for you to have made it through all that information, for it means that you're ready to start putting your plans for health, diet, and growth into action. It means you should now be ready to go it on your own.

As you've been processing this information and learning all that Intermittent Fasting has to offer, you likely now have a strong and firm sense of what this dietary & lifestyle shift can do for you, and it's time to start putting all that information and all that knowledge into motion in your life.

The next step will be to make a few changes, but they don't have to be big ones! Start by just skipping the next meal! Go a day with a little less in your food portions! Begin your adjustment period into Intermittent Fasting without fear or concern, for it will be much easier and much more worthwhile than you could ever have imagined.

I am eager to hear what successes you all experience after reading this book, so please feel free to write about what happens by way of an Amazon review! You can also leave any general feedback on this book in an Amazon review, and I'd be equally appreciative. Thank you for your time and all your hard work getting ready for the Intermittent Fasting shift in your life! I can't wait to see what the future holds for you now.

Form new Mini Habits, Increase Longevity, and Burn fat Forever with the Best solution to a Paleo or Keto Diet! (complete Weight Loss Guide, Intermittent Fasting tips)

By
Serena Baker

Introduction

Congratulations on downloading *"Mediterranean Diet for Beginners,"* and thank you for doing so. By starting this book, you have shown an interest in changing your life for the better, and you should be applauded for this decision.

The following chapters will discuss everything you need to know to successfully begin incorporating the Mediterranean diet and lifestyle into your daily life. You'll find that there is so much more to this eating plan than food, though! The Mediterranean diet is a relaxed, low-stress, active, and social way of approaching life. By celebrating fresh, local, and whole foods, the people who inspired this diet have taught us that dieting does not have to make us feel like we are depriving ourselves of anything. You'll learn to feed yourself in a way that genuinely fuels your body from the inside out in a way that makes you feel alive and satisfied.

In this guide, you'll learn about the solid scientific research that went into the establishment of the Mediterranean diet, as the number one diet for long-term healthy living. You'll discover how to start approaching life as the Mediterranean people do, and how to begin shopping for food with a new perspective.

Finally, you'll also learn how to lose weight on the Mediterranean diet, and you'll get helpful hints for if you are having trouble losing weight. You'll even get a good breakdown of many of today's popular fad diets, from ketogenic to intermittent fasting. You'll learn how the Mediterranean diet stacks up against each one and how to compromise between this eating plan, and any others that are beneficial for you. This guide concludes with 20 mouth-watering and healthy Mediterranean recipes to get you started on your new way of life. Every effort was made to ensure it is full of as much useful information as possible. So please, enjoy!

Chapter 1: The Mediterranean Way of Life

An incredibly diverse group of countries encompasses the Mediterranean Sea. These countries include, but are not limited to the following: Italy, Morocco, France, Syria, Spain, Greece, and Egypt. Because there are so very many countries in this region, it is impossible to define a single "diet" that includes cuisines from the whole region. Instead, the Mediterranean diet contains the commonalities of these areas: namely, efforts to eat copious amounts of vegetables and fruits, whole grains, lentils, beans, fish and shellfish instead of meat, and plenty of olive oil. These components make up the heart of the Mediterranean eating plan.

The Philosophy Behind the Mediterranean Diet

The Mediterranean diet is not just another diet fad. Instead, it's a whole way of life – a way of life millions of people residing along the Mediterranean Sea have been thriving on for thousands of years. This lifestyle incorporates an array of flavorful and healthy ingredients, along with a different approach to life than the one to which most residents of the United States have become accustomed. There is so much more to the Mediterranean diet and lifestyle than just food. It's also about making small changes to your daily life that improve the overall quality of your health.

Reducing Stress

By and large, people living in Mediterranean countries tend to have less stress in their daily lives when compared to their American counterparts. They spend much more time enjoying meals with loved ones. They often relax and take a short nap after lunch. It's common to take a 2-hour break in the middle of the day to have lunch and take a nap. When scientists looked into this practice of a post-lunch rest, they realized that the people in this area have a good thing going. Recent research showed that regularly snoozing for a short time in the middle of the day reduced your risk of death from heart disease by 37 percent!

The Effects of Stress

Doctors often neglect to counsel patients on the impact of chronic stress on long-term health during routine exams and office visits. This gap in information given to patients is unfortunate, since stress may be the most critical health risk factor faced by most of us! The issue with stress is that we cannot measure it in the same ways that we measure blood pressure or heart rate. It is a somewhat ambiguous and subjectively measured factor, especially since what causes stress for one person may not cause stress for another. Some people thrive on certain types of stress, like the pressure of looming deadlines and a fast-paced work environment. However, if one of those same people was to decide to start a family and have her first child, she might find herself overwhelmed by an entirely different type of stress. On the other hand, certain people seem like they are born to handle the everyday pressure of raising children, with all its unpredictability and sleepless nights; but if they suddenly entered a fast-paced work environment, they might lose their minds entirely.

No matter the source, chronic stress causes an increase in cortisol and adrenaline, which are stress hormones. These hormones are responsible for the rise in blood pressure. It also raises one's heart rate, making the formation of blood clots in the process. Research has proven that heart attacks are more likely to occur in individuals who face chronic stress. Moreover, certain people who are highly reactive and impatient are even more prone to cardiovascular problems.

Daily Exercise

Besides lower stress levels in the Mediterranean culture, exercise is also part of everyday life. People do a lot of walking – and who wouldn't, with the beautiful weather and stunning views around the Mediterranean Sea? Whether it's waking up early to take a stroll, walking to the grocery store, gardening, or sweeping the yard, physical activity isn't given a second thought.

Family Time

The family is a big part of the Mediterranean culture. Family get-togethers aren't just during the holidays or special events in this culture. They're held every few days or at least once a week, creating a special bond among everyone at the table.

Chapter 2: The Mediterranean Diet in a Nutshell

In summary, the Mediterranean diet is a way of eating that combines whole non-processed foods and is rich in a wide variety of health-promoting vitamins and nutrients. Countless health and dietary experts recognize it as the ideal nutritional plan for long-term heart health and weight control – in fact, multiple clinical trials have demonstrated its benefits.

Many people who live along the Mediterranean coast don't think of their eating habits as a diet – it's just their way of life. Eating fresh, plant-based ingredients and getting regular physical activity is how they've lived for thousands of years.

There's no subscription to prepackaged Mediterranean diet meals you can buy, and there isn't a calorie meal plan you have to follow. You don't have to ban any food group, and you don't have to avoid carbs. Instead, you'll be more conscious and mindful of how you eat every day – just like the millions of people along the Mediterranean Sea.

How the Mediterranean Diet Became Popular

This way of eating was first brought to light by American scientist Dr. Ancel Keys. In the late 1950s, Keys conducted the Seven Countries Study, which followed the diet and lifestyle habits of participants in seven different countries – the Netherlands, Finland, Japan, Yugoslavia (formerly), Italy, and the United States.

Keys' findings showed that eating habits, types of fat consumption, and physical activity greatly decreased the study participants' risk of cardiovascular disease. What's more, it highlighted the fact that the people who had already embraced this diet and lifestyle lived along the Mediterranean Sea. Since Keys' work, hundreds of other studies have been conducted and continue to support his findings of the many benefits of the Mediterranean diet. You'll read more about the research of Keys and other scientists in Chapter 3, "Who Should Consider the Mediterranean Diet and Why?

Not every single country along the Mediterranean eats the same way, but most do embrace many aspects of the Mediterranean diet as part of their culture and way of living. The type of food consumed differs based on country, culture, agriculture, and even regions within each country. This section of the book will give you an understanding of the essential parts of this diet.

Below the key components that combine to make this diet and lifestyle work:

- Eating fresh, in-season fruits and vegetables
- Reducing processed foods
- Using whole grains in everyday recipes
- Using "good" fats or unsaturated fats, from fish, extra virgin olive oil, nuts, and avocados.
- Eating moderate amounts of low-fat dairy such as Greek yogurt, which has lots of probiotics that are great for your digestive system, and cheese.
- Consuming lean protein from eggs, fish, poultry, and small amounts of red meat.
- Filling your diet with legumes, including beans, seeds, and nuts
- Using fresh and dried herbs and spices to boost flavor
- Drinking red wine, in moderation (This isn't necessary if you do not consume alcohol.)
- Getting daily exercise
- Reducing your stress level
- Making time for family

The above are some basic things to remember, but what's most important is to incorporate each item in a way that suits you, so you're more likely to continue to follow these tips.

Creating a Mediterranean Table

Adapting your mindset to the Mediterranean diet certainly will be an adjustment if you are accustomed to how we typically approach food in the United States. In the Mediterranean diet, you'll encounter smaller portion sizes and get used to the idea of eating less meat overall defines a serving size. You'll also find that Mediterranean meals often include several dishes of equal importance, rather than the main dish with a few sides. The following recommendations can help guide you as you work to incorporate the main principles of this diet into your daily routine!

A New Approach to Your Plate

Usually, you might decide on a protein around which to center your meal. Next, you add a couple of vegetable or starch dishes to go with this protein. Instead of this approach, try starting with one or two vegetables and making the protein an equal contributor, instead of the main event. It's not that you will be making more food; you will just need to approach the composition of the meal a little differently.

Moderation is Essential

Regardless of the types of food you consume, it is essential to make sure you monitor the portion sizes. Portions are noticeably smaller within the Mediterranean diet, and the yields of the recipes in this book reflect that concept. You may be used to serving just four people with a pound of pasta, but you should try to stretch it to serve at least six. Additionally, a piece of chicken or meat for one person should be around five ounces. Sorry, but you are not likely to encounter a 10-ounce steak on this diet! A Mediterranean lunch or dinner is made up of appropriately-sized contributions from a few different dishes.

Eating Fresh and Local Foods

Much of Mediterranean meal planning focuses on maximizing vegetable and fruit consumption. Additionally, participants in this way of life celebrate seasonality by purchasing the product that is in season. Sticking to in-season produce helps you ensure that you get the freshest products possible. There are some canned and frozen versions of vegetables available year-round, of course. These include canned fava beans, frozen corn, canned tomatoes, and jarred artichoke hearts.

You'll find very little processed food on this diet. What you will discover are far more flavor and far fewer preservatives and sodium. Many of the dishes are brought to life by using herbs and spices instead of other, not-so-good-for-you ingredients. This diet is thousands of years old, dating to a time when you couldn't find all types of fruits and vegetables available 365 days a year like you can today. People ate what was in season. This practice is excellent because in-season produce has more nutrients than when it's out of season.

Buying local products also helps ensure you get the freshest ingredients. Fruits and vegetables lose nutrients the longer they sit in the refrigerator, so buying from local growers lets you know what you're getting is freshly picked and still contains many beneficial nutrients. But when fresh isn't available, people along the Mediterranean have learned to preserve food without using high amounts of salt, sugar, or fat, by drying beans and grains and drying and pickling vegetables.

Another key to the Mediterranean diet is that although about 35 percent of your caloric intake comes from fat, it is from *monounsaturated fats* – or healthy fats from olive oil, nuts, avocados, and fish. Nuts are a large part of the Mediterranean diet and contribute to your protein intake as well. Incorporating a handful of nuts every day can help boost your protein, omega-3 fatty acids, good fats, vitamin E, and fiber while reducing cholesterol.

Daily Consumption of Whole Grains and Beans

Since Mediterranean inhabitants eat red meat and poultry sparingly, their major sources of protein include beans, lentils, nuts, and whole grains. These components can be featured in soups, stews, and salads. They also round out more filling dishes when combined with a source of protein, like fish. Additionally, they can enhance dishes that feature pasta or vegetables. Whole grains contribute many essential nutrients like antioxidants, but not all Mediterranean grains are whole grains.

Consume Less Red Meat and More Seafood

The consumption of fresh fish and shellfish, has been a way of life in the countries along the Mediterranean Sea since men first started casting their fishing nets in that body of water. The benefits of eating seafood include their low-calorie count and high levels of heart-healthy polyunsaturated fats. Sardines and mackerel are included in the more affordable types of fresh fish. Fish can be prepared in many healthy ways including pan-roasting, broiling, grilling, and baking.

Using Meat for Flavoring

Since red meat is typically expensive, it has been a common practice in the Mediterranean region to combine it with more economical ingredients, like beans or grains. That way, less meat is used overall. Those who practice this diet as a way of life implement this idea by creating dishes that highlight meat along with a central vegetable or grain. They may make use of more flavorful cuts of meat, so even a small portion of meat has an impressive effect.

Serving Fruit for Dessert Instead of Sweets

Throughout the Mediterranean, fruit is often served as a dessert. Cakes and cookies are only eaten during special occasions, not every day. To try and lower the amount of saturated fat when you do serve sweets, you can try replacing all or part of the butter in your desserts with olive oil. Sometimes, to still produce a satisfying sweet that is worthy of serving to guests, you will need to keep some of the butter in the recipe. This idea may require you to do some experimentation as you endeavor to pursue this healthier way of eating and living.

Variety is the Spice of Life

Mediterranean meals are full of diversity, so try serving dishes with a range of different temperatures and flavors. The idea of serving some foods cold helps make meal planning easier since some things can be made in advance or even served as leftovers. As you discover more and more dishes that fit into this eating plan, you'll find it is easy to mix and match recipes.

The Mediterranean Diet Pyramid

In the 1990s cooperative work between nonprofit health and cultural food organization called "Oldways", and the Harvard School of Medicine led to a visual representation of the diet. This image was the 1993 creation of the Mediterranean Diet Pyramid. The visual representation of this way of eating serves as a handy tool for anyone interested in trying the diet. It essentially symbolized the results of the Seven Countries Study by Ancel Keys. One of his most important findings was that people who lived on the island of Crete, had lower rates of heart disease than the other study participants. Keys attributed this fact to their diet, which was full of vegetables, grains, and legumes and simultaneously low in saturated fat. The Mediterranean Diet Pyramid ultimately helped make the diet popular in the United States. In 2008 the Mediterranean diet pyramid received some minor updates, and the result is the version described here.

Like the old USDA food pyramid of the 1990s, the Mediterranean Diet Pyramid places different types of foods in differently-sized spaces which represent their relative importance in this eating plan. The most common elements of Mediterranean meals, along with the plant products, form the base of the Pyramid. These include herbs and spices, nuts, olive oil, fruits and vegetables, whole grains, legumes, and beans. It is recommended that people following this diet base every meal on the foods in this large bottom space.

On the next level Pyramid, you will find seafood. Fish and shellfish should be consumed at least twice weekly. Further up are poultry and eggs, along with dairy products. These foods are eaten moderately in daily or weekly servings. At the very tip of the Mediterranean Pyramid are red meats and sweets, which are consumed in relatively small quantities and least often.

Off to the side of the Pyramid (or, in some versions, occupying a small space under meats and sweets) is red wine, which is safe to consume in moderation under this eating plan. When it comes to red wine, "moderation" generally means no more than one to two (5-ounce) glasses each day.

Additionally, the Pyramid contains a side reminder to hydrate by drinking plenty of water. You don't often see water in a food pyramid, but it's an integral part of any diet and lifestyle. More than half of your body is composed of water, making it a very integral part of nutrition. Drinking water is an important habit to develop as you exercise, too, because it helps boost your metabolism. You should focus on drinking plain water instead of sodas or sugary fruit drinks that could be filled with high fructose corn syrup. If you struggle with drinking enough plain water, try adding some fresh fruit or herbs to your glass to change the flavor.

Finally, in most versions of the Pyramid, another base piece consists of the essential components of the Mediterranean lifestyle: daily exercise, enjoying meals with others, relaxation, and smoking cessation.

Recommended Servings and Serving Sizes

Although the Mediterranean diet pyramid doesn't go into a lot of details about how many servings and the serving sizes of each food group are recommended, there are some guidelines that dietary experts can agree on. The following guidelines should help you get an idea of how much of each food group in this diet you should try to eat, and what constitutes a serving size:

- **Whole Grains**: Four to six servings recommended each day.

    Serving Size: ½ cup cooked grains such as oats, quinoa, or pasta, or 1 slice of bread.

- **Vegetables:** Four to eight servings recommended each day.

    Serving Size: 1 cup raw or ½ cup cooked veggies.

- **Fruits:** Two to four servings recommended per day.

Serving Size: ½ cup of fresh fruit or 1 average piece of fruit or ¼ cup dried fruit.

- **Beans and legumes:** One to three servings recommended each day.
  Serving Size: 1/3 cup dried or 1 cup cooked.

- **Seafood:** Two to three servings recommended each week.
  Serving Size: 4 to 6 ounces.

- **Fats:** Three to six servings recommended each day.
  Serving Size: 1 ounce of nuts or seeds (the number of nuts in an ounce depends on the size) or 2 tablespoons of groundnut or seed butter. For oils, a serving size is one tablespoon.

- **Herbs/Spices/Condiments:** Herbs can be used in large quantities. For condiments, aim for one tablespoon per serving. Salt should be reduced to 1 to 2 teaspoons per day.

- **Poultry:** One to three servings recommended each week.
  Serving Size: 3 to 4 ounces (should fit in the palm of your hand).

- **Red Meat:** No more than three to four servings recommended each month.
  Serving Size: 3 ounces

- **Eggs:** Three to four servings recommended per week (but egg whites can be eaten daily).
  Serving Size: 1 whole egg

- **Dairy:** One to three servings recommended per day.
  Serving Size: 1 cup of yogurt or 1 ounce of cheese; aim for low-fat or nonfat versions.

- **Alcohol:** Aim for no more than one to two drinks per day.
  Serving Size: 4 ounces of wine or 12 ounces of beer.

- **Sweets:** Avoid these and try to opt for one serving of fruit instead of other sugars.

In the case of the food groups in which a range of servings is recommended, use your common sense about your body size and activity level. If you are a tall, muscular person who gets a lot of physical activity, you can probably aim for the upper limits of serving sizes. For example, you could probably safely eat three servings of dairy per day, four servings of red meat per week, and six servings of healthy fats per day. Conversely, if you are a small or inactive person, or if your goal is to lose weight, you should try to eat the lower number of servings recommended for each food group. For more information about weight loss, see Chapter 5: "The Mediterranean Diet and Weight Loss."

Chapter 3: Who Should Consider the Mediterranean Diet and Why?

This chapter delves into the Mediterranean Diet's many health benefits. If you find that you are attracted to these benefits or discover that it may be suitable for a specific health problem you currently face, you should certainly speak with your physician about adopting this eating plan.

Let's start by looking at the main parts of the Mediterranean Diet and their primary health benefits!

The Main Parts and Health Benefits of the Mediterranean Diet

Whole Grains

Whole grains are a vital part of the Mediterranean diet, and research has shown that consuming them decreases the risk of deadly diseases like diabetes and cancer, not to mention heart disease. A single whole grain kernel consists of an outer layer, called the bran (containing fiber); a middle layer (containing complex carbohydrates and protein); and an inner layer (including vitamins, minerals, and protein). Refining grains, a process that is common in the United States, leaves only the middle layer of the grain. This destruction of the most nutritious layers results in grains that do not have the vitamins and fiber known for fighting diseases. A few examples of whole grains you might use on this eating plan are kasha, barley, oatmeal, and farro.

Full of fiber, vitamins, minerals, and complex carbohydrates, whole grains present your body with numerous benefits. They aid digestion; decrease cholesterol levels, assist with weight loss because they keep you full longer; and help prevent deadly chronic diseases that are associated with poor cardiovascular health and high blood sugar. Whole grains are essential to people who have diabetes because they help regulate blood insulin levels.

Fresh Fruits and Vegetables

Farmers' Markets in the Mediterranean region are typically full of fresh, in-season, locally-sourced fruits and vegetables. These natural foods contain high levels of vitamins, minerals, complex carbohydrates, and fiber that reduce the risk of cancer and heart disease, among other ailments. Phytonutrients, which are found at high levels under the skins of these plant products, are strong components that help us fight life-threatening health issues.

Fruits are easy to incorporate into your daily diet plan. You can buy fruit that's easily transportable, like apples, bananas, peaches, or apricots. Dried fruit is another great option. It's easy to pack and take with you, it won't spoil, it has an intense flavor, and most of the nutrients are retained. Fruits are also a great addition to your meals. Try adding dried fruit or pomegranate to salads, enhance the flavor of chicken with figs or dates, or add fresh fruit to a cup of Greek yogurt for a snack filled with protein and nutrients!

Fruits also contain natural sugars, which are easier for your body to digest and provide more nutrients than refined sugars. Natural sugars found in fruits are often called fructose. Although you've been trained to fear the word "sugar" and associate it with something terrible, naturally occurring sugars are essential for the body.

Now for vegetables. These good-for-you foods are another cornerstone of the Mediterranean diet. Vegetables are full of fiber, vitamins, minerals, chlorophyll, potassium, carotenoids, flavonoids, and antioxidants. They're also low in fat, sodium, and cholesterol. With the Mediterranean diet, vegetables should be at the base of every meal and should take up half your plate. They are very low in calories, so eating a lot of vegetables can be very beneficial – they'll fill you up with all the right nutrients, with nothing extra!

Nuts

These tasty little morsels, like walnuts, pine nuts, and almonds, are full of heart-healthy monounsaturated fat, and they have long been a vital component of the Mediterranean diet. Because of their high fiber and protein level, nuts can help people lose weight because they help people who eat them to feel full for longer periods. They are also good sources of several key vitamins. Research has shown that eating nuts regularly is linked to lower risks of heart disease and heart attack and to lower cholesterol levels. Plus, nuts' fiber and antioxidants help your digestive system and slow cell aging.

However, nuts are high in calories, so eat in moderation. A handful a day can go a long way. Also, in a way, nuts are like vegetables: if you douse them with salt, sugar, and chocolate, you end up losing all the benefits they offer. So, skip the add-ons, and reap the rewards!

Beans (Legumes)

Beans are also consumed regularly as a part of this diet. They contain high levels of fiber, which increase satiety and reduce cholesterol levels. Beans are also important sources of protein and vitamins. The fiber associated with regular bean consumption has been linked with a lowered risk of life-threatening issues like heart disease, cancer, and diabetes.

Fish

Oily fish, prevalent in the Mediterranean diet, provide us with essential protein and omega-3 fatty acids. Omega-3 fatty acids have a favorable impact on cholesterol and triglyceride levels and help lower our risk of heart attack. They also help to reduce inflammation and, with regular consumption, decrease the risk of sudden death due to fatal cardiac arrhythmias.

The two omega-3 fatty acid types that you may have heard of in fish are *EPA (eicosapentaenoic acid)* and *DHA (docosahexaenoic acid)*. EPA is a fatty acid that prevents blood clotting and helps reduce pain and swelling. Its presence in your diet helps regulate and avoid issues like heart disease, Alzheimer's disease, personality disorders, depression, high blood pressure, and diabetes. DHA improves brain function, helps thin blood, and lowers triglyceride levels. It also reduces the risk of type 2 diabetes, heart disease, neurodegenerative diseases like dementia, and attention deficit hyperactivity disorder (ADHD).

A warning about fish: Several species of fish may contain high levels of mercury, and other contaminants, so pregnant women and young children should be careful. However, for most adults, the heart health benefits of fish consumption are much greater than the risks. To minimalize any risks, look for fish that contain the lowest mercury levels. The best choices are salmon, albacore tuna, herring, sardines, shad, trout, flounder, and pollock. It is best to avoid swordfish, shark, king mackerel, and tilefish because they usually have the highest mercury content.

Olive Oil

Olive oil, made directly from olives that have been crushed and pressed, is the heart and soul of this eating plan. It provides much of the rich and distinctive flavor from the Mediterranean region, and it contains seemingly endless nutritional benefits. This oil is monounsaturated fat, which means that it boosts cardiac health. It also contains polyphenols, antioxidants, and omega-3 fatty acids. These vitamins and minerals help lower cholesterol while reducing our chances of developing diseases like cancer, heart disease, arthritis, osteoporosis, and even type-2 diabetes.

Using olive oil regularly instead of butter or margarine helps reduce your risk of heart disease, inflammatory disorders, cancer, and diabetes. Consuming olive oil also helps lower levels of bad (LDL) cholesterol while keeping or improving healthy levels of good (HDL) cholesterol.

Olive oil can assist with weight loss. A Boston study demonstrated that an eating plan that included regular consumption of nuts and olive oil led to sustained weight loss over a year and a half. This eating plan was compared to a low-fat diet. People also stayed on this olive oil- and nut-rich diet for a longer time because of these foods' satiety.

Red Wine

Moderate alcohol consumption has been shown to help reduce our risk of developing heart disease. Red wine in particular, often part of a Mediterranean meal, is believed to have several advantages over other forms of alcohol. Red wine consists of polyphenols and resveratrol, both of which promote cardiac health. Resveratrol is an antioxidant that helps maintain healthy levels of cholesterol and also contributes positively to blood clotting. It is present in higher levels in red wine than white.

It's critical to remember that alcohol should only be consumed in moderation. A person's daily wine consumption should not exceed one or two (5-ounce) glasses per day. For people who prefer to avoid wine, grape juice is an excellent alternative. Grape juice – specifically purple grape juice – also significantly reduces the risk of heart attack.

Target Health Conditions of this Diet

You likely picked up on several health conditions that may receive benefits from components of the Mediterranean diet, but not all of them were included in previous descriptions. Below is a list of diseases or health conditions that can be improved or prevented by following a Mediterranean-based eating plan:

- Cancer
- Depression
- Dementia
- Diabetes
- High Blood Pressure/Stroke
- Heart Disease
- Metabolic Syndrome
- Obesity

Focusing on Heart Disease

Many books and experts who talk about the Mediterranean diet focus almost exclusively on its benefits in heart disease prevention and overall contributions to heart health. The reason for this focus is simply that cardiovascular disease is the number one killer worldwide. Here's a rough breakdown of the eight most common ways people died in 2010 in the U.S.:

- Heart disease: 600,000 deaths
- Cancer: 575,000 deaths

- Recurring lower respiratory diseases: 140,000 deaths
- Stroke: 130,000 deaths
- Accidents: 120,000 deaths
- Alzheimer's disease: 85,000 deaths
- Diabetes: 70,000 deaths
- Kidney disease: 50,000 deaths

At a glance, heart disease and cancer death seem comparable. However, when you look at deaths caused by cardiovascular disease – which is responsible for heart disease but also affects the entire circulatory system – they number more than 800,000. This includes heart disease, stroke (90 percent are the clotting type related to the very same process that causes heart attacks), and many other blood-vessel-related conditions. Diabetes, Alzheimer, and kidney disease are also thought to be linked to or worsened by cardiovascular disease. Cancer is number two on the list, resulting in around 575,000 deaths. However, of those, 160,000 cases are lung cancer, in which the majority are related to smoking. The next most common cancers are colorectal (50,000 deaths per year), breast (40,000), pancreatic (40,000), and prostate (30,000). Each one of these cancers can be caused by a combination of many different factors – such as genetics, diet, environmental toxins, hormones, and various other carcinogens. Cardiovascular disease, in contrast, has a more unified cause, so following its prevention plan has the potential the help most people's greatest risk. Furthermore, the same diet and lifestyle recommendations that help prevent heart and cardiovascular disease generally help protect from cancer – and all the other major chronic diseases – as well.

A History of Research Behind the Mediterranean Diet

The pursuit of an ideal diet began in earnest when heart attacks began increasing at an alarming rate in the 1940s. No health concern was more urgent than heart disease at that time, as it was responsible for around 40 percent of the total deaths in the United States (and if you included stroke, which is related to the same disease process, the figure was 50 percent). The overall death rate was much higher then as well, and a disease of the arteries caused about half the deaths. Again and again, men and women in the prime of life were dropping from sudden cardiac death. It wasn't long before the leader of the United States, President Dwight Eisenhower, had a massive heart attack at the age of 65, while still in office. The nation was on edge and looking for answers.

Evidence that the Mediterranean way of eating can be beneficial to people who suffer from cardiovascular disease, and other conditions was ultimately discovered in some independent and widely-publicized research projects and clinical trials. Here, we'll look at some of them:

The Seven Countries Study

Previously mentioned in the description of the Mediterranean Food Pyramid, this landmark twenty-year study by Dr. Ancel Keys was able to show that a diet that contained low levels of saturated animal fat and processed food was linked to a low incidence in mortality from coronary heart disease and cancer. Diet had been suggested as a probable cause for heart disease since at least the turn of the century, but an understanding of the connection remained murky at this point. Cholesterol had been identified as a likely candidate for having something to do with it, singled out because it was found that the arterial clots themselves were full of it. When some substantial studies came out demonstrating that cholesterol levels in the blood were higher in patients with heart disease, many thought they had at last confirmed the dietary culprit. However, Keys performed studies that showed it was not the cholesterol one *ate* that made it available in the blood to form blockages in the arteries.

Keys had begun to hypothesize what else it might be other than cholesterol in the diet that was causing those high levels when an unusual patient took him in a new direction. A sick farmer was referred to him by a medical school in Wisconsin. After trying various treatments, Keys checked the farmer's blood cholesterol level, and the first reading was sky high – 1,000 mg/dL, compared with the national average of 220 or 230. The man's brother had come in with him as well and had a reading of 600. The two were sent to Keys' Minnesota lab, where they stayed and were fed an almost fat-free diet for a week. After a week, their cholesterol levels had both dropped by about 50 percent. Keys wondered what might happen if he gave them some fat. When he gave them food with saturated fat in it, the cholesterol levels of both men increased dramatically. Hence, it appeared that it was *fat* that was affecting their cholesterol levels. It was ultimately the result of this particular investigation that led to his painstaking testing of how fats, in their many forms, could affect health and disease.

Keys went on to perform further feeding studies, which convinced him that, indeed, blood cholesterol levels were the result of how much fat was consumed in the diet. Postwar statistics also revealed an intriguing clue to the mystery. Keys noticed that some of the wealthiest, and probably best-fed, people in America suffered from significantly high incidences of heart disease. However, in postwar Europe, where supplies of food like meat and dairy were quite low, heart disease rates had declined. He was also impressed and intrigued by the alleged low rates of heart disease being reported in the area around the Mediterranean Sea. Ultimately, upon invitation from an Italian colleague, he left for Italy in 1952.

From a research standpoint, Keys' stay in Italy was the dawn of collecting international health and nutritional data to compare with other regions. For example, it quickly became clear to him that cholesterol levels in Naples were much lower than those being measured in America and England. It also soon became clear as he toured Italian hospitals that heart disease in this region was indeed a rarity. From here, Keys continued to expand his research, collecting data from Madrid, Spain as well. His reports stimulated an international group to join in, generating measurements and diagnoses in South Africa, Japan, and Finland.

The collective data supported the notion that differing fats in the diet were associated with varying blood cholesterol levels, as well as in the frequency of heart disease. In Japan, for example, they observed communities with a low incidence of heart disease who ate a very low-fat diet, whereas in Finland they encountered hard-working men, many of whom were quite physically fit by outward appearances. However, in this land of butter and cheese, many of these apparently fit men suffered from heart disease.

Keys observed and followed the lifestyle patterns in Naples, where he was staying. He became enamored with the food and culture of southern Italy. Keys absorbed and embraced the people's culinary tastes and habits, their tendency to walk everywhere and get out in the sunshine, their tendency to drink a glass or two of wine with supper. This seaside introduction to the culture of Naples turned out to be just as important as the scientific revelations to come. He found that the diet of this region was loaded with fruits, vegetables, and whole grains. The way of eating here was also different from certain other diets in that it contained significantly fewer dairy and meat products and offered fewer sweet baked goods for dessert. These observations culminated in his development of the Seven Countries Study.

With the active participation of leading international cardiologist Paul Dudley White (President Eisenhower's cardiologist), the study was a meticulously planned and executed ten-year investigation of the epidemiology of coronary disease in sixteen populations of six Western countries and Japan. Around 13,000 men were studied, aged forty to fifty-nine, from Japan, Greece, the Netherlands, Finland, Yugoslavia (formerly), Greece, and Italy. It took years of negotiations, fundraising, planning, and trial run before communities began being monitored in 1958. This massive endeavor was a milestone study on numerous counts, marking the first effort in history to leap international borders and compare diet-disease associations between communities with widely differing culinary and lifestyle populations. The hope was that the regional differences in risk, health behavior, and biological factors could be measured, thus providing direction to prevent – or at the very least decelerate – heart disease around the world.

The first results from the Seven Countries Study were published in 1970, after ten years of data collecting. As Keys had predicted, a high amount of fat in the diet – especially saturated fat – was correlated with heart disease. Both the island of Crete in Greece and southern Italy were heralded as the shining stars of the study, having by far the lowest proportion of heart disease and the longest life expectancy. Americans, by contrast, had a 72 percent greater chance of dying from heart disease than the Italians. It was clear that diet was related, but since only the macronutrient contents were used for analysis (that is, the amounts of proteins, carbohydrates, and fats), the specific foods of the diets were not published for some time.

The Seven Countries Study generated much interest in the eating habits of the healthiest people in the world. Over time, more research was published that demonstrated the benefits for the other elements of the Mediterranean diet aside from eating little saturated fat. It turned out that all the antioxidants, vitamins, minerals, fiber, healthy proteins, complex carbohydrates, and wine these people were consuming promoted health and longevity as well.

Throughout the 1980s and 1990s, scientists, nutritionists, and doctors worked to define what the Mediterranean diet precisely was. After all, there are more than fifteen countries that surround the Mediterranean Sea, with overlapping cuisines. Which formula was the best? In the end, they kept coming back to the 1960s rural diets of Crete and southern Italy. Also, in 1989, one of the directors involved in the Seven Countries Study published a historical record of what the subjects in all the countries under investigation were eating around the time of the study. The proportions for Crete and southern Italy at that time are now taken to be the ideal healthy Mediterranean diet, because of those communities' very low incidence of various diet-linked conditions (though their diets and disease rates have since changed). Other investigations confirmed the data and thus constituted the principal research basis for the proportions of foods in modern Mediterranean diet pyramids.

The Lyon Diet Heart Study

One of the first clinical trials in support of the therapeutic benefits of the Mediterranean eating plan, a groundbreaking study known as the Lyon Diet Heart Study, came in 1994. Six hundred patients in France who had had heart attacks were randomly assigned to either a Mediterranean-style diet, or a control diet similar to what the American Heart Association recommended for the reduction of heart disease risk. Two years into the study, the compelling results came in: the Mediterranean group had a 73 percent reduced risk of coronary events, and 70 percent reduced overall chance of dying as compared with the control diet. The study was meant to go for five years but was stopped after an interim analysis showed such significant beneficial effects in the patients receiving the Mediterranean diet. Adding to the significance of this study was the intriguing finding that, despite a robust connection between adhering to the Mediterranean diet and living longer, no significant associations were seen for the individual components of the diet. It was becoming clear that it was the diet as a whole that was best for your overall health, and protection from disease.

As research continued, it also became apparent that the Mediterranean diet was not just better for your heart. Any condition related to arteries or veins generally benefitted. Data from a series of studies have also shown that sticking to the Mediterranean diet is can help lower the risk of developing various cancers. The risk of contracting degenerative diseases of the brain such as Parkinson's and Alzheimer's appears to be cut as well. Moreover, the Mediterranean diet has long been recognized to reduce mortality overall.

Below is a summary of several other scientific investigations that contributed to the evidence pointing to the Mediterranean diet's myriad health benefits:

The DART Study

In this research project, over 2,000 men were studied to test whether the polyunsaturated fat in seafood would help protect against heart disease. The results showed that eating a modest serving of oily fish twice per week reduced the risk of heart disease death by 32 percent and overall mortality by 29 percent.

The Alzheimer's Disease Study

Dr. Nikolaos Scarmeas, from New York's Columbia University Medical Center, showed that a Mediterranean diet was linked to a 68 percent lower chance of developing Alzheimer's disease. He led another study that demonstrated that eating a Mediterranean food helped Alzheimer's disease patients to live longer, healthier lives even after their initial diagnosis.

The Singh Indo-Mediterranean Diet Study

This trial placed 499 patients who were at risk for heart disease on a diet that was full of foods derived from plants. The study found that the diet change reduced incidences of heart attack and sudden cardiac death. Researchers also discovered that the subjects had fewer cardiovascular events, overall than those on a conventional diet.

The Metabolic Syndrome Study

Dr. Katherine Esposito and her Italian colleagues tested the effects of a Mediterranean diet on patients who suffered from metabolic syndrome (a condition that is characterized by obesity, elevated blood pressure, unhealthy cholesterol profile, and indications of vascular inflammation). The Mediterranean diet improved all the symptoms of metabolic syndrome.

The Spain Study

This Spanish study compared a Mediterranean diet to a diet that was low in fat. Although planned for a longer period the study abruptly ceased after just 4.8 years, because of the those following the Mediterranean diet showed a massive 30 percent reduction in significant cardiovascular incidents (i.e., heart attack, stroke, death). In the *New York Times* on March 2, 2013, medical experts stated that for the first time in history a diet had been proven to be as effective as drugs in preventing cardiovascular complications, including death.

Recent Thoughts About the Mediterranean Diet

By the year 2000, the quantity of fat in the Mediterranean diet came under scrutiny, challenging many deeply held beliefs that a low-fat diet was the ideal. It was acknowledged that, even though high amounts of fat in the diet were linked to heart disease, some of the regions the Mediterranean diet were modeled after actually had a high-fat content in their food, up to around 40 percent of their daily calories. But it wasn't saturated fat they had been eating – their diet had olive oil poured all over it. With a combination of monounsaturated fat and antioxidants that benefit health in numerous ways, olive oil seemed to be an essential health elixir, helping to thwart disease in many shapes and forms.

An interdisciplinary, multicultural conference was held in Rome to further update and standardize the Mediterranean diet in 2005. The participants invoked an ancient Greek word, *ataraxia* – which connotes "equilibrium," "lifestyle," and being in a state of robust tranquility while surrounded with trustworthy and affectionate friends – to accompany the description of the Mediterranean diet. In presenting it as more than just a diet, they recognized the importance of the entire lifestyle upon health and well-being. Physical, social, and culinary activities also play an essential role.

Unfortunately, scientists still have not found a magic bullet for health, probably because one does not exist – our bodies are far too complicated for that. However, at this point, we seem to have identified the diet of the people who have the least disease and live the longest. Perhaps the magic is that the Mediterranean diet improves universal biological features that promote health, such as reducing inflammation and excess body fat; maybe it's the environment of warm social connection enjoyed by the healthiest communities; maybe it's that a diet so fresh, varied, and delicious, yet simple, is so easy to take on. It is most certainly partly all these things.

Who Should Consider Switching to the Mediterranean Diet?

The answer to this question seems pretty straightforward. Anyone who wishes to pursue ideal cardiovascular health and consequently do all they can to prevent death by diet- or lifestyle-related complications should consider the Mediterranean diet! In other words, experts have presented a strong case for the idea that this eating plan is ideal for just about anyone!

Possible Socioeconomic Limitations

However, research published in 2017 showed that the benefits of this diet might be limited to people of higher income status, higher socioeconomic backgrounds, or who are more "educated". Specifically, researchers found that advantages to heart health from the Mediterranean diet may be limited to only top socioeconomic status groups.

The reasons behind these findings could be several different things. First, it is possible that the higher quality of food available to the upper socioeconomic classes is responsible for the benefits of this diet. Additionally, a more extensive variety of food is available to those at a higher income level. Finally, it is highly possible that those with more education were able to adhere to the diet more closely and recall their adherence with better accuracy. In other words, perhaps not everyone reported their strict following of the menu with perfect recall. Because many possible details that influence how well people report their eating habits, this research is not necessarily accurate or reliable.

Does this study mean that those of us who earn lower incomes or did not pursue education after high school, should throw up our hands and give up all hope of benefitting from a Mediterranean diet? Of course not! It just means that everyone, regardless of income, background, or education level, needs to commit firmly to the eating plan if they wish to reap its rewards. No one is expecting perfection, but what matters is that we all make small and continual strides towards improvement.

Additionally, it is possible that those of us who earn lower incomes may face more significant challenges when it comes to finding high-quality ingredients. However, it is possible to follow the Mediterranean diet on a limited budget. In general, whole, unprocessed foods are more affordable than their more processed counterparts. Fresh fruits and vegetables, especially when locally sourced, are usually economical. Canned light tuna in water has just as many health benefits as fresh salmon. There are many affordable whole grains, and poultry is generally budget-friendly. Since red meat and dairy are eaten in limited quantities, these items should not impact your bank account too much.

As far as more expensive items, like olive oil, herbs, and spices go, it is suggested that you purchase these things in limited quantities anyway. If you have too much of any of these items on hand, you run the risk of them spoiling before you can use them. In the next chapter, you'll see the most commonly used spices and herbs, so you'll get an idea of where to start. Additionally, it is suggested that you start with just what you need for the first few recipes you plan to make, and then build slowly from there. There is also a buying guide for olive oil!

Those with Food Allergies and Sensitivities

It is true that the Mediterranean diet includes several components that are highly allergenic to some people, including certain nuts, shellfish, dairy, and products that contain gluten. However, even those people can follow this eating plan with a few adjustments!

For those who are allergic to shellfish, dairy, or nuts, there are plenty of options for protein and unsaturated fats in this diet, so you should be able to follow it while making the necessary substitutions. You have likely already become accustomed to making these changes in your diet, so these adjustments are not likely to be very difficult for you.

For people who have gluten allergies or sensitivities, there is no reason that you cannot follow this diet as well. Those who have not researched the Mediterranean diet sometimes incorrectly assume that it is full of bread and pasta. However, at this point in the book, you should understand that there are many other integral parts to this diet which do not contain any wheat or gluten whatsoever. Additionally, many whole grains do not contain gluten, like the following: amaranth, buckwheat, corn, millet, most whole oats, rice, sorghum, and wild rice.

Also, quinoa, although technically not a grain, can be consumed similarly to grain, and it does not contain gluten. If you have been diagnosed with gluten intolerance, like Krone's disease, or gluten sensitivity, you are likely already used to making gluten-free substitutions and adjustments to your diet. You can rest assured that the Mediterranean diet is not off-limits to you!

REMINDER: Always Consult Your Doctor!

Regardless of your physical fitness, health concerns, or food allergies, it is always strongly recommended that you consult your healthcare provider before changing diets or beginning a new exercise program. Your doctor can address any underlying concerns that may make it necessary for you to pursue a particular variation of the Mediterranean diet. He may recommend that you undergo specific testing before making any dietary changes or after following a new diet for several months.
In the next chapter, you'll learn how to start making the necessary steps towards incorporating the Mediterranean diet and mindset into your lifestyle.

Chapter 4: Getting Started

Changing your eating habits to follow the Mediterranean diet can be very exciting. Knowing that you're making the conscious decision to improve your diet – and your life – in a positive way and eat healthier is the first step of the Mediterranean diet. It might seem overwhelming at first, but you don't have to make all the changes in one day. The more small changes you make, the more benefits you'll see, which will inspire you to make more beneficial changes. Those benefits will pay off big in the long run – for you and your family.

Keys to Embracing the Mediterranean Lifestyle

To successfully incorporate this new way of eating into your life, you should seriously consider adopting other parts of the Mediterranean lifestyle as well.

Reduce Your Stress Level

Remember the discussion of the dangers of stress in Chapter 1? One of the most critical keys to revamping your lifestyle to fit your new way of eating is *stress reduction*! This instruction may be a tricky one; after all, we all have periods of stress in our lives. Additionally, some of us seem destined to have more pressure in our lives than other people. Regardless, handling stress should begin with trying to find a realistic perspective on the factors that cause our stress, then doing what we can to change those factors. Maybe you can't really follow the Mediterranean habit of taking a 2-hour midday break, but you can incorporate ways to reduce your stress throughout your day. First, a physical exercise program will help tremendously in stress reduction, simply because research has shown that active people can handle pressure better. There is an explanation for the beneficial effects of exercise on stress levels: People who engage in regular aerobic exercise have lower adrenaline levels that rise less dramatically in stressful situations.

Try to get some physical activity every day. It can be something as casual as walking your children to the park or walking your dog for 20 minutes while enjoying nature instead of looking at your phone. If you can't do something physical, try preparing a cup of coffee or tea, disconnecting from technology, and sitting on your porch to relax and sip it for 20 minutes. It's the little things that allow your body and mind to rest.

In addition to a regular exercise program, some form of relaxation practice such as meditation, yoga, or self-hypnosis can also help reduce your overall stress level. If all these lifestyle changes do not result in a significant reduction in stress, then consider a consultation with a psychologist or psychiatrist.
Below are ten practices for you to try for stress reduction:

- Daily exercise
- Meditation
- Prayer
- Enjoying close relationships with friends and family
- Setting realistic goals in life
- Living within your (financial) means
- Yoga
- Enjoying interests and hobbies outside of work
- Having an optimistic outlook on life and never losing your sense of humor
- Laughing, smiling, and enjoying your life!

Exercise Daily

Although this recommendation was mentioned under stress reduction, it bears further investigation. Daily exercise is a very important part of the Mediterranean lifestyle, and it does more than help you handle stress. Whether it's walking to the market or working in the garden (two common forms of daily exercise in the Mediterranean region), regular daily exercise is essential for good health. Activity raises good (HDL) cholesterol, lowers blood pressure and optimizes bone health, which reduces the risk of osteoporosis. Regular exercise also promotes a healthy sense of well-being; no wonder why there are so many healthy and happy senior citizens in the Mediterranean region of the world!

Lack of exercise, along with poor food choices, has contributed to the recent outbreak of American obesity. Additionally, several studies have shown that being out of shape physically is more detrimental to our health than just being overweight. Sadly, we have become a nation of "couch potatoes," and getting people to adopt a habit of exercising is difficult. We like using the elevator instead of the stairs; we park as close as possible to the store; we ride in carts instead of walking through a nine-or-18-hole game of golf!

The solution is to begin incorporating exercise into your daily activities. You do not need to start with anything ridiculous by jogging 5 miles a day or biking for an hour every morning. Just walking for thirty minutes a day can significantly decrease the risk of heart attack or other cardiovascular problems. Additionally, a regular exercise program will reduce fatigue and improve your lung function. If you add resistance training with light weights, your bone health will improve further, and you'll be helping to maintain your muscle tone.

It's up to you to decide what physical activity you enjoy, figure out how you can make it a part of your life, and stick with it until it becomes a habit. You can integrate many different forms of exercise into your daily life. Among of which are walking during your lunch break, walking the kids to the park instead of driving, going for a bike ride on Saturday morning instead of watching cartoons, walking between stores instead of driving when you're out shopping, or playing a sport the entire family can enjoy. If you have children, you can set an example that physical activity should be part of their lives as well.

Here are some more easy tips for incorporating exercise into your life:
- Walk in place for thirty minutes while watching TV.
- Park farther away from your office, grocery store, etc. and enjoy a short walk through the parking lot.
- Walk for the first part of your lunch break, before you eat.
- Use a pedometer and aim to get 10,000 steps each day.
- Choose to take the stairs for a change.

Physical activity is an indispensable part of the Mediterranean diet, and order to be successful with adopting this eating plan, you must integrate exercise into your life as well as making healthy eating choices.

Family Time

In the fast-paced and highly technical era we live in, it's sometimes hard to make time for family. However, it should be a priority. Try planning dinner times so everyone can sit and eat a meal together. It helps build relationships and connections. Much research has shown that people with strong family interaction are less likely to suffer from depression.

If you don't live near any family members, you can create the same atmosphere with friends. Try planning weekly or bi-weekly get-togethers and maybe having a different friend host it each time. Making meals potlucks takes the stress off any one person preparing a big meal. When you go, take a Mediterranean diet recipe to share with your friends!

Other Tips for the Mediterranean Way of Life

Besides reducing your stress level, getting more daily physical activity, and increasing your family time, the following are solid guidelines that you should consider beginning to incorporate into your new way of life. Remember, no one is expecting you to make dramatic changes overnight. You can start each of these guidelines with baby steps, then work your way into more significant changes:

- Eat a variety of fresh, whole foods
- Limit intake of fat, except healthy sources of unsaturated fat
- Avoid refined sugar
- Avoid excessive salt
- Limit portion size
- Consume alcohol only in moderation (preferably red wine)
- Hydrate by drinking plenty of water!
- Laugh, smile, and enjoy life – never lose your sense of humor.
- No smoking! If you do smoke, take steps to begin quitting today.
- Relax a little every day (especially after meals, if possible)

A Fresh Look at Your Kitchen

Stocking your kitchen is so important when adopting a new way of eating. You do not want to be left with a pantry empty of healthy foods, and only chips or a boxed cake mix as your meal or snack options. Keeping a well-stocked pantry gives you more alternatives and ideas of dishes you can make. Experimenting with different herbs, spices, and flavors is also important because these are low-calorie and fat-free ways of adding a tremendous amount of flavor to any dish, all completely guilt free.

While you will be using lots of familiar ingredients like chicken, salmon, quinoa, and chickpeas in the Mediterranean diet, you should also investigate less familiar ingredients and research recipes for grains like barley, beans like chickpeas, meats like oxtails, and fantastic seafood like monkfish. Depending on how in-depth you wish to pursue this way of eating and living, you may want to learn to work with finicky ingredients like grape leaves and phyllo dough and flavor builders like sumac, preserved lemons, and pomegranate molasses.

This book only has 20 recipes, which is just a small start to an infinite number of other equally-healthy dishes that you can find through research. Below is information about core kitchen ingredients you may want to begin stocking. It is not recommended that you buy all the spices, herbs, condiments, and other long-lasting ingredients at once. To do so would be extremely costly! Instead, decide on the recipes you want to try first, and begin your shopping list with the ingredients necessary for those dishes. Eventually, you'll find that your pantry and refrigerator are well-stocked with ingredients from each of the following categories:

Fresh Fruits and Vegetables

Fruits and vegetables are a large portion of the Mediterranean diet food pyramid, so let's look at them first. When purchasing these foods, it's best to buy items that are in season, when they're at their peak flavor. Buying produce in season, and as close to the time it was picked, ensures you get fruits or vegetables with the most nutrients. One way to ensure you're getting fresh produce is to buy from local farms and farmers' markets. It's also a good idea to smell produce before you buy it. If it smells great, it's likely to taste great, too.

Here are some critical fruits in the Mediterranean diet: Apples, apricots, avocados, bananas, berries, dates, figs, grapes, melons, olives, peaches, pomegranate, and strawberries.
The following are some of the vegetables that are popular on this diet: Artichokes, beets, bell peppers, carrots, cauliflower, dandelion greens, eggplants, garlic, leafy greens, onions, potatoes, romaine lettuce, tomatoes, and zucchini.

You may have noticed that tomatoes are on the vegetable list. Technically, tomatoes are a fruit, not a vegetable. But because most people recognize them as a veggie and prepare them like they would other vegetables, they are listed with the other vegetables here. Tomatoes and tomato products are a huge part of the Mediterranean diet, from fresh tomatoes to tomato sauce, tomato paste, and so much more.

Many recipes in this book, and from the Mediterranean region, include garlic and onions. These two ingredients can provide an abundance of flavor to any dish. They're versatile and can be cooked in different ways to alter their flavors and pungency, too. For example, when onions are sautéed slowly, they give off a sweet taste, and when garlic is toasted in olive oil, it has a nutty flavor. Both can also be used raw atop a salad or in a dressing.

Also, in the recipes, you'll see how often vegetables are easily integrated into the recipes and prepared in so many different ways. But remember that vegetables on their own are very healthy, so don't load them with heavy creams or sauces that add lots of calories and fat. And keep in mind that the more vegetables you eat, the more your body benefits. So work them into your meal plan as often as you can.

Canned and Dried Beans

Legumes are an integral protein in the Mediterranean diet – in fact, they help make up the most extensive section of the menu, along with fruits, vegetables, and whole grains. Legumes can be eaten green or harvested and dried for their beans or seeds. This group includes chickpeas, fava beans, lentils, peas, and white beans. They can be eaten alone or also prepared as a part of a recipe with other ingredients. Two examples might be whole-wheat spaghetti with lentils or shrimp with white beans.

Canned beans typically work well in salads, sautés, and soups. You may consider using dried beans in recipes that take a longer time to cook, such as stews. In these dishes, cooking the beans can help develop the flavor more completely. Some people like to prepare dried beans by brining them; this preparation helps them to keep their original shape during the cooking process. Fava beans are one of the only beans that are more frequently used fresh than dried or canned, although preparing fresh fava beans is somewhat labor-intensive.

Legumes and their seeds are very inexpensive, and when dried, they last a long time. These ingredients are prevalent in Mediterranean countries because they store easily and can be used throughout the winter, when traditionally the availability of meat or vegetables was low. Rehydrating them is very simple – just soak in water for a few hours and cook as desired. You can also rehydrate them, cook them in water, and freeze the cooked legumes. Then, when you're craving hummus, you can just defrost the beans in minutes, rather than a few hours. Using dried beans is also a great alternative to using canned goods which can sometimes have many preservatives.

Grains

Grains, including rice, are central to many Mediterranean dishes. There are different ways to cook each type of grain. For example, farro should be boiled in an excessive amount of water, but rice only needs just enough boiling water to absorb it all fully. You should strive to have at least 50 percent of the total grains you eat be whole grains. As mentioned previously in this guide, refined grains contain far fewer beneficial nutrients and can even negatively impact your risk of developing diseases like diabetes.

Some of the many examples of whole grains include bulgar, corn, oats, barley, brown rice, buckwheat, farro, freekeh, spelt, wheat berries, whole rye, whole-wheat flour, and wheatberries. Quinoa, although it is actually a nutty-flavored seed, can also be placed in this category because it's commonly thought of as a grain and is typically prepared and eaten in the same fashion as other grains.

Whole grains are incredibly versatile. You can use them in soups; prepare them as pilafs; work them into bread, cakes or cookies; or even use them as a stuffing. It's simple to make any dish a bit healthier by replacing all-purpose flour with whole-wheat flour, for example. Or replace long-grain rice with brown rice and regular pasta with whole-wheat pasta.

Pasta and Couscous

Pasta is an essential part of many Mediterranean dishes, but it is frequently prepared in ways that are not familiar to most American home cooks. For example, some pasta dishes get their distinctive flavors from strong spices like cinnamon or cloves. Heartily robust whole-wheat pasta should be a nice change from the typical pasta to which most Americans are accustomed. Couscous is commonly eaten in North Africa as a part of many diverse dishes, and it is sometimes served on its own. Residents of the eastern part of this region use a type of couscous called pearl couscous, which has larger grains and is toasted instead of dried.

Olives and Olive Oil

Olives are quite well-known for their role in Mediterranean food. Many types are crushed and pressed to make olive oil, but others are grown exclusively for eating. If your grocery store has a refrigerated section with olives, those are more highly recommended than the canned and jarred types, since the preservatives in those make them very salty. If you have enough food preparation time, experts even suggest that you purchase olives that still have the pits, then remove the pits from them yourself.

You will learn more about olive oil in a different section of this chapter.

Fresh and Dried Herbs

Herbs and spices were added to the pyramid representing the Mediterranean diet in 2008 because they are such an essential component of this diet. They add an abundance of flavor without extra calories or fat. They also add some vitamins and minerals to your diet. And they're long-lasting: dried herbs and spices often stay good for at least a year when stored in an airtight container.

Some recipes call for fresh herbs, while others call for dried. Why the difference? Flavor. The flavor of fresh herbs can be very earthy and pungent, while dried herbs are nuttier and toned down. You can add fresh herbs to recipes without needing to cook them, whereas dried herbs more than likely need to be prepared to bring out their flavor.

The dishes of the Mediterranean region are flavored by a wide variety of fresh herbs, such as basil and mint. Many proponents of this diet grow these herbs themselves, while other people purchase them from stores or farmer's markets. In the recipes of this book, fresh herbs are used as a garnish for some recipes, but they contribute to the main flavors of other dishes. Most fresh herbs will not last long in storage, but with proper handling, you should be able to keep them for a week or so. First, you'll need to rinse them carefully, then dry them as thoroughly and as gently as possible. Then roll them in paper towels, but keep the rolls loose. The last step is to place the roll of herbs and paper towels in a bag with a zipper seal and keep it in your refrigerator.

You should also strive to keep plenty of different dried herbs available because many Mediterranean recipes call for them. Blends of various herbs are a terrific way to add complex flavor to dishes. Dried herbs lose their flavor 12 or fewer months after you open the container. You can test them for their freshness by rubbing a pinch of one between your fingers. If you do not detect that herb's signature aroma, you should discard it and buy a new supply. Some herbs that you purchase fresh can be dried in the microwave, but this should only be attempted with the heartier herbs, like rosemary and thyme.

Here are some common herbs in the Mediterranean diet: Basil, bay leaf, cilantro, marjoram, mint, oregano, parsley, rosemary, sage, and thyme.

Mediterranean Spices and Spice Blends

The various cuisines in the Mediterranean region can typically be distinguished from each other by the spices that are used in the recipes. You may already have some of the spices you'll need, like cinnamon and paprika. Other spices, like sumac and Aleppo pepper, will be less known to you. Spice pastes and dry blends are also frequently used to add distinctive flavors to dishes: Examples include *za'atar*, a favorite eastern Mediterranean blend; North African *ras el hanout*; and *harissa*, a North African chili paste. You can purchase these and other spice blends at some supermarkets or grocery stores, but if you are unable to find them at the store, you can learn to make your own with a little practice and research.

Storing your spices at a safe distance from heat and light will help you keep them longer. You should pay attention to the smell and appearance of each spice; when either of these characteristics changes, it's probably time to throw it out. When buying spices, you'll find that the better brands are usually pricier, but the difference it makes in your recipes is often well worth the extra cost. Additionally, a little spice goes a long way, so the price isn't so bad if you consider how many meals you can get out of one small bottle of any spice.

The following are common spices used in Mediterranean cooking: Allspice, black pepper, cayenne, cinnamon, cloves, coriander, cumin, dried ginger, paprika, sumac, and zaatar.

Salt

Salt enables you to get the most flavor from a dish. That's why you'll see salt called for in almost every recipe in this book. You can use table salt, which is the most common type, or you can use sea salt instead if you like. Sea salt has more minerals and is an organic salt, while table salt, on the other hand, is more processed. And don't worry about the sodium content of these recipes. The tiny dashes of salt you'll be adding only increase the sodium minimally. The high levels of sodium that are detrimental to cardiovascular health, are found in processed foods that contain vast quantities of salt-laden preservatives to extend the shelf life of the product.

Cheeses, Cured Meats, and Nuts

Just a little bit of cheese, like feta; cured meat, like pancetta; or nuts can add a lot of flavor to Mediterranean recipes. For example, some dishes are flavored with just a little bit of salami or prosciutto, while many kinds of pasta and salad dishes need only a tiny sprinkle of Parmesan cheese to round out their flavor.

Nuts are standard in the Mediterranean diet. They're tasty on their own or in many sweet or savory dishes. Whether roasted, toasted, or raw, walnuts, pine nuts, almonds, pistachios, sesame seeds, peanuts, cashews, and other nuts are full of flavor. They are frequent additions to salads and other side dishes. Additionally, some seasoning blends include nuts as an important component. Some of the recipes later in the book demonstrate how easily you can add nuts to your diet.

Although the recommended intake for dairy is only two servings per day, still opt for low-fat versions because dairy products are high in saturated fat. Avoid processed cheeses and instead choose fresh cheese made of sheep's or goat's milk. These are usually more flavorful, and a little goes a long way.

When you plan to store cheese in the refrigerator for more than a few days, you should wrap it first in parchment paper, which lets the cheese breathe. The top layer over the parchment paper should be aluminum foil. This impenetrable layer keeps the cheese from drying out and also keeps out unwanted flavors from other refrigerator inhabitants. For long-term storage of nuts, keep them in your freezer; otherwise, you run the risk of them becoming rancid. To bring out the flavor of nut in recipes, try toasting them in the microwave or on the stovetop before incorporating them into dishes.

Fresh Meats, Poultry, Eggs, and Seafood

The Mediterranean diet includes many types of meats, including beef and lamb, poultry and eggs, and seafood, providing much-needed protein in small serving sizes.

Beef, lamb, and goat are conventional in the Mediterranean region, although they are eaten in limited quantities. When purchasing red meats, opt for the leanest cuts. Fillet, although it's costly, is an excellent cut of red meat because it's tender and very lean. You can grill it without adding any fat and can season with fresh or dried herbs and spices to enhance the flavor. For ground meat, whether it's beef or lamb, aim for 95 percent lean and 5 percent fat ground. The small amount of fat helps keep the meat moist and flavorful. Adding spices can also boost the flavor.

Poultry and eggs are other great sources of protein. Chicken, duck, turkey, and fowl are usually quite affordable and can be prepared in many different ways. To eliminate a lot of saturated fat when cooking poultry, remove the skin. And if you're looking for a piece of leaner meat, use the breast. The recommended portion of poultry is 1 (6- to 8-oz) serving every 2 days.

Over the years, eggs have developed an unfortunate reputation for being high in fat and cholesterol, but when you're on the Mediterranean diet, you should have no reason to avoid eggs. This eating plan recommends that you eat up to 7 eggs per week. They are a top source of high-quality protein and are still low in calories.

Seafood is an excellent option for those who don't like poultry or red meat. It contains a lot of protein but is low in fat and calories, and it contains many different vitamins and minerals. When purchasing seafood, it's recommended to buy fresh fish from a good source – preferably someone who has a high volume of customers, so you know the fish hasn't been sitting in the display case more than 2 days. If the fish smells terrible, it will taste bad too, so don't buy it. And skip any cooked fish displayed next to raw fish to avoid cross-contamination. If you can't find fresh fish, your next best option is frozen. Just make sure that you cook it right away after defrosting it.

Condiments

Yogurt: It may surprise you to hear that yogurt can be a condiment, but it's frequently used that way in this eating plan, where a small scoop can be a topping. It can also be incorporated into sauces and poured over some dishes. You'll find that some recipes you encounter in your new Mediterranean style of eating require the richer flavor of whole-milk yogurt, but you can use low-fat or nonfat yogurt in some dishes. Greek yogurt, which is thicker and creamier than regular yogurt, is typical in Mediterranean countries – and around the world. It contains live and active bacteria that aid your digestive and immune systems. Greek yogurt can be an ingredient or a side dish to many breakfast, lunch or dinner recipes. This type of yogurt, in particular, is perfect for making thick and creamy Tzatziki sauce, which can be used as a dip or sauce for dishes like kebobs, gyros, and falafel.

Tahini: This paste is made from ground sesame seeds. It can be included as a topping by itself or incorporated into certain sauces and dips, like hummus and baba ghanoush.

Pomegranate molasses: This thick, syrupy condiment, made by simply reducing pomegranate juice, is used to add tang to many dishes. If you cannot find it in a store, it is easy enough to learn to make it on your own.

Preserved lemons: This little-known ingredient comes from North Africa. It is very easy to make preserved lemons, but they take several weeks to cure. Once cured, you can keep them for up to six months in the refrigerator without worrying about them spoiling. However, if necessary, you can make a quick substitute: Combine four 2-inch strips of lemon zest, minced, 1 teaspoon of lemon juice, ½ teaspoon of water, ¼ teaspoon of sugar, and ¼ teaspoon of salt. Microwave this mixture at 50 percent power until the liquid evaporates, about 1 ½ minute, stirring and mashing the lemon with the back of a spoon every 30 seconds. This method makes about 1 tablespoon of a preserved lemon substitute.

Dukkah: This condiment stems from Egypt. It consists of a combination of spices, seeds, and nuts, and it can be used to add a distinctive flavor to many dishes. It can also be simply added to olive oil to be used as a dip for bread. Not all forms of dukkah are the same. As you become more comfortable with preparing Mediterranean cuisine, you may find that you prefer to make your own dukkah.

Honey: Honey is a natural sweetener that's superb for use in baked goods, desserts, breakfast, teas, and coffee. It contains 70 to 80 percent monosaccharides, fructose, and glucose, which give it its sweet flavor. Research has shown that the antiseptic and antibacterial properties of honey can help with a cold or heal wounds.

Waters: Have you ever had orange blossom water or rose water? Neither has a substantial nutritional value, but they both have intense flavors and add an exotic flavor element to any dessert or drink. You can find them at specialty food stores. They're fairly inexpensive.

Syrups: Syrups in Mediterranean cooking are most commonly used for desserts, as a topping. Simple syrup, for example, is made from simmering sugar, water, a bit of lemon juice, and a flavoring such as orange blossom water or rose water. Then you can drizzle it on phyllo pastries, fruit, or yogurt to sweeten.

All About Olive Oil

Perhaps the most significant ingredient of Mediterranean cuisine is olive oil. Only produced from crushed and pressed olives, there may be no other food product that is quite so distinctive to this eating plan than this one. Olive oil is classified according to grades that indicate its quality. The highest quality is called "extra-virgin," and this is the type that should be used for all of your cooking and raw applications of olive oil in this eating plan. Its flavors vary wildly depending on which olives were used for producing it and how ripe they were at harvest time. It is made in several parts of the Mediterranean; however, California is also a top producer of olive oil in North America.

You may remember that olive oil helps support the goal of incorporating more healthy unsaturated fats into your diet. The use of this fat instead of butter or margarine is far healthier for your heart. Additionally, since it is a food derived from a plant, it contains antioxidants and other essential nutrients that help your body fight diseases like cancer and diabetes.

Extra-virgin olive oil is known as an important component of dressings and a tasty dip for pieces of bread. On top of those well-known uses, it is also often drizzled over vegetables and pasta, incorporated into sauces for meats and fish, and used for cooking ingredients of soups and stews. For a heart-healthy application in desserts, try replacing butter with olive oil in pastries. For example, a pie or tart crust made from olive oil can have a surprisingly savory flavor and tender texture.

Buying and Storing Olive Oil

Finding the right extra-virgin olive oil for your cooking purposes can be confusing. Unfortunately, standards for olive oil quality are typically voluntary and rarely enforced, so the bottles labeled "extra virgin" may be a company's lower-quality olive oil that is being passed off at a higher price than it deserves.

Extra virgin olive oils range wildly in price, color, and quality, so it's hard to know which to buy. While many things can affect the style and flavor of olive oil, the main factors are the variety of olive and the time of harvest (earlier means greener, more bitter, and pungent); weather and processing also play a part. The best-quality olive oil comes from olives pressed as quickly as possible without heat. The use of heat in pressing the olives coaxes more oil from the olives, but it sacrifices the excellent taste of the product.

Since there is a vast number of different types of extra virgin olive oils for sale on grocery store shelves, some of the experts at America's Test Kitchen took it upon themselves to try and narrow down the options for confused consumers. They came up with a plan to find the best "everyday" extra virgin olive oil and the best "high-end" product so they could confidently recommend specific products.

To find the best "everyday" olive oil, the test participants tasted 10 lower-priced olive oils in various applications. The testers also sent each of the oils to a lab to be evaluated for quality and accuracy of grading. Finally, they had 10 highly-trained olive oil tasters for their opinion on each variety.

Ultimately, one oil was the clear winner over the other "supermarket" brands: California Olive Ranch Everyday Extra Virgin Olive Oil. They discovered that this product's superiority could be attributed to this company's vigilance and control over quality and speed in every step of production. Since olives change flavors rapidly after they are picked, speed is highly relevant in getting from picking the olives to pressing them into oil, then quickly bottling the oil before it oxidizes and spoils. At $9.99 for a 500 mL bottle, it is more expensive than some inferior oils found in the grocery store, but it is much more economical than the high-end oils.

It may surprise you to discover that the most expensive high-end oils are not always the best ones. The high-end oil that came out on top for America's Test Kitchen is called Gaea Fresh. This oil was produced in Greece, and at $18.99 for a 500 mL bottle, is surprisingly affordable when compared with other "high-end" olive oils. Tasters were impressed by this oil's flavor, which was strong but well-balanced. It is recommended that you use this high-end oil in raw applications only, where strong flavor counts.

Of course, you're bound to find countless other opinions about which is the best olive oil for your cooking needs. As you grow more experienced in using and tasting olive oil, you may even come up with your favorite brand of extra virgin olive oil. Feel free to experiment and research to your heart's content!

Keeping Your Olive Oil Fresh

Three criteria will help you decide on the quality of your extra-virgin olive oil before purchasing it and help you keep it as fresh as possible.

Oil Origin: Bottlers, often print where their oil has been sourced from on the label; look for oil that has been sourced from a single country.

Harvest Date: Even though some oils may have a "best if used by" date, the harvest date is a more accurate descriptor of its freshness. Typically, olive oil starts to degrade about a year and a half after the olives were harvested. You'll want to buy a bottle that has the most recent date, and certainly one within the last year. If there is no harvest date, it may not be a good idea to buy that bottle at all. Since olives are harvested during the fall and winter in the Northern Hemisphere, you may only be able to find bottles that list the previous year.

Dark Glass: Only dark glass adequately shields the oil from damage caused by light and air. Clear glass and clear plastic just do not have what it takes to keep your olive oil as fresh and pristine as possible.

To Store

You should never keep your olive oil out where it will be exposed to light. Since it is a plant product, it contains chlorophyll, which will oxidize in sunlight. Additionally, make sure not to keep your olive oil where it will be exposed to unnecessary heat, such as a cabinet right next to the oven. It is best kept in a cool, dark cabinet, but not in the refrigerator, where it will become cloudy and thick. Once you open a bottle of olive oil, you need to use it within three months, but an unopened bottle can be kept for up to a year.

You only need your sense of smell to check your olive oil for its freshness. Pour a little of it out and smell it. The smell of rancid olive oil tends to remind people of either stale walnuts or crayons. If this is the smell that greets you, it's time to throw the bottle out.

Now that you've learned how to begin making the necessary changes for embarking on this new phase in your life, it's time to look specifically at how the Mediterranean diet can help you in your weight loss goals if that is your desire.

Chapter 5: The Mediterranean Diet and Weight Loss

The Mediterranean diet – a well-balanced diet that includes healthy fats and complex carbohydrates – offers the best alternative to popular fad diets if you're looking to lose weight without sacrificing your health. By pairing this eating plan with lower stress and increased exercise, you can do more than just lose a few pounds; you can also reduce your blood pressure, cholesterol, and blood sugar. As you've already read in earlier chapters of this book, those are just the beginning of the benefits.

One of the essential influence's diets can have upon health is by merely establishing weight control. Being overweight can damage every system in the body and is a risk factor for all our most serious, debilitating diseases. The Mediterranean diet helps one maintain a healthy weight by providing complex carbohydrates, fiber, and protein to help you feel full and to slow digestion, so you feel satisfied for longer.

People who live in the Mediterranean region *and* follow a Mediterranean diet and lifestyle, are leaner than their American counterparts for the following reasons:

- Exercise is a part of their everyday lives.
- They consume foods with high fiber content, like fruits, vegetables, beans, nuts, and whole grains. These foods lead to high satiety, the feeling of being full.
- They avoid trans fats, which are associated with weight gain and obesity. Instead, they eat healthy fats, like monounsaturated fat and omega-3 fat. Fat consumption,

in the form of olive oil, nuts, and fish, also leads to satiety.

- They consume complex carbohydrates rather than simple carbohydrates, and they avoid refined sugars, which are linked with obesity. Complex carbohydrates also help the consumer feel full longer.
- Food is not "super-sized" in Mediterranean countries like it is in America. It is the quality of food, not the quantity of food, that makes a good meal!

Calories and Weight Loss

The secret to weight loss is simple: burn more calories than you consume. Quite simply, Americans consume too many calories! We eat large meals and then a snack in the evening while we sit and watch TV. This excessive caloric intake combined with our sedentary lifestyle is the reason that obesity is a significant public health threat. Although the Mediterranean diet is not one that is geared towards obsessive calorie-counting, there are several tips you can follow that will help you reduce your overall calorie intake, without having to write down every calorie you put in your mouth.

Portion Control

We must learn to eat smart. First, we need to limit the portions of the food we eat. Over the years, restaurant portions and packaged food portions have gradually increased in size. The average bagel now weighs four to five ounces (equal to four or five slices of bread), cookies are the size of saucers, and an order of pasta in a restaurant would once have fed a family of four. To determine what an "average" serving of packaged food should really be, check the nutrition label. You may be surprised to learn that the "single" packaged food portion you've been assuming was for one is actually intended for two – or more.

You don't need to weigh or measure foods, but use common sense, and learn to eyeball right portions. For instance, a medium orange is about the size of a tennis ball, and a three-ounce piece of meat is about the size of the palm of your hand.

In Chapter 2, you read the recommended serving sizes and number of servings in each of the Mediterranean diet's food groups. As suggested in that chapter, you can use your body size, activity level, and weight loss goals as guides to the number of servings you should have within the guidelines. If you stick to these recommendations, you may be able to lose weight without counting a single calorie. However, if you have trouble losing weight by merely controlling portions and number of servings, you can learn more about counting calories later in this chapter.

Increased Physical Activity

Besides learning to limit our portions, we also need to start exercising. In chapter 4 you read several tips on slowly incorporating more physical activity into your life. If you struggle with motivation, try to remind yourself that you are doing this for more than just your waistline – it's essential to exercise if you wish to live as long and as healthy of a life as possible. By starting and maintaining a habit of daily exercise, you'll help ensure that you'll be around to enjoy life with your family and friends for as long as possible.

Another tip for increasing your motivation to exercise is to find someone who will help you remain accountable. Finding a workout buddy not only helps you when you struggle to get off the couch and get active, but it also adds elements of fun and social interaction to your exercise routine.

More Whole Foods, Fewer Processed Foods

Finally, we must also replace processed food, refined sugar, trans fats, and saturated fats with healthier, lower-calorie whole foods – as in the Mediterranean diet. Also, because the concentration is on fresh food, you're not eating commercially-made products that are higher in calories as well as designed to compel you to overeat and create irresistible cravings. It's also easy to follow because it doesn't involve an extreme diet makeover, and – as you'll see when you start trying recipes – it tastes so good!

Counting Calories

As previously stated, the Mediterranean diet is not one that necessarily lends itself to obsessive calorie counting. Ideally, you'll find that by focusing on eating fresh and whole foods, limiting portion size, avoiding processed foods, and increasing your activity level, you will begin to lose weight naturally. However, if you find that the scale won't budge, or you reach a "plateau" in your weight loss – a point at which your weight loss stalls and you can't lose that last 10, 20, or 30 pounds – it may become necessary to begin counting calories, at least until you become accustomed to estimating your body's nutritional needs.

Determining Your Metabolic Needs

The first step towards learning how many calories you should be consuming to lose weight, is to figure out your basal metabolic rate, or BMR. This amount of energy (in calories) that you would burn if you were sleeping all day long. Below are the steps for figuring out this equation:

1. Determine your weight in centimeters. You can either measure it in centimeters or, if you know how tall you are

in inches, multiply this number by 2.54. For example, if you are 63 in. in height, multiply that by 2.54, and the answer is approximately 160 cm.

2. Determine your weight in kilograms. You can get your weight in pounds and convert it to kg by dividing it by 2.2. For a 135-pound person, you would divide 135 by 2.2 for an answer of about 61.4 kg.

3. If you are a male, use this equation to get your BMR in calories per day:

> BMR = (cm of height multiplied by 6.25) + (kg of weight multiplied by 9.99) − (your age multiplied by 4.92) + 5.
> With the above numbers, if you are 36 years old, the equation would look like this:
> BMR = (160 x 6.25) + (61.4 x 9.99) − (36 x 4.92) + 5 = 1000 + 613.39 − 177.12 + 5 = 1441.27 calories per day

4. If you are a female, use this equation to get your BMR in calories per day:

> BMR = (cm of height multiplied by 6.25) + (kg of weight multiplied by 9.99) − (your age multiplied by 4.92) − 161
> With the above numbers, if you are 36 years old, the equation would look like this:
> BMR = (160 x 6.25) + (61.4 x 9.99) − (36 x 4.92) − 161 = 1000 + 613.39 − 177.12 − 161 = 1275.27 calories per day

Next, you need to use your BMR and daily activity level to determine your total energy expenditure (TEE) per day or the amount of energy (in calories) your body burns each day at your current activity level. The BMR result is multiplied by a factor that is used to estimate your physical activity level (PAL) to determine their TEE, as follows:

- If your lifestyle is sedentary or includes only very light activity, such as working in an office, multiply your BMR by 1.53.

- If your lifestyle is active or moderately active, such as standing work in a factory, housecleaning, or if you get a moderate amount of daily exercise, multiply your BMR by 1.76.

- If your lifestyle is vigorously active, with extremely strenuous physical labor or intense and lengthy daily exercise, multiply your BMR by 2.25.

For example, for the woman with the BMR of 1275.27 calories per day above, let's say she has a moderately active job. She would multiply 1275.27 by 1.76 to get approximately 2,244 calories. This is the approximate amount that this woman needs to eat each day if she wishes to maintain her current weight of 135 pounds.

Determining Your Weight Loss Needs

If you are trying to lose weight, the only way to do it is by consuming fewer calories than you burn. There are two ways to do this – either you can incorporate more vigorous physical activity into your daily life and keep eating the same number of calories, or you can decrease the amount of calories you eat per day. You can choose to do both, but you must be vigilant to make sure you aren't making too many drastic changes. If you end up in a situation in which you are consuming drastically too few calories for your body's needs, you can end up with serious health complications. At the very least, your body might go into "starvation mode," in which it conserves every precious ounce of energy in a desperate attempt to stay alive. In this case, you may not end up losing as much weight as you had hoped. The key is to strike a balance, in which you have enough of a calorie deficit to lose weight, while still consuming enough energy to fuel your body adequately.

The safest way to determine how many calories to cut is by using math once again. A wise and safe strategy in weight loss is to try and lose 1 to 2 pounds per week. The loss of one pound requires a deficit of 3,500 calories. Spread out over a week, and that makes a deficit of 500 calories per day. You could either try to exercise enough to about 500 calories of extra energy each day, eat about 500 fewer calories daily, or strike a balance by cutting 250 calories and burning an extra 250 calories.

For example, with the same example woman who weighs 135 pounds and needs to eat 2,244 calories each day to maintain this weight. Let's say she wishes to lose about one pound per week until she reaches her goal weight of 120 pounds. To accomplish this, she has three options:

1. She could maintain the same activity level and eat 1,744 calories each day for a daily calorie deficit of 500.
2. She could find a daily activity that burns an extra 500 calories each day, while still consuming 2, 244 calories each day.
3. She could eat 1,996 calories each day and find an activity that burns an extra 250 calories each day.

With any of the three above options, the woman ends up with a weekly reduction that totals 3,500 calories, which should lead to a weight loss of about a pound each week.

Help with Counting Calories

Each recipe in this book reports an accurate calorie count per serving, along with protein, carbohydrates, and fat content. There are only 20 recipes to get you started here, but you can find an infinite number of Mediterranean diet recipes on the internet and in other books once you are ready to start trying more dishes. Many of these recipes will also include calorie counts.

If you want to try a recipe that does not report calories, use common sense and compare it to other similar recipes. Or you can get incredibly detailed and calculate the calories of the entire recipe by adding all the ingredients together and dividing the total by the number of servings.

There are a lot of phone and tablet apps that will help you keep track of your calories and encourage you when you meet your goals each day. You can also do internet searches on calorie counts for different foods and meals, and you will often find remarkably accurate results.

If the Scale Still Won't Budge – Troubleshooting

In some cases, you may feel like you are doing everything right and *still* not losing weight. Or perhaps you started off with rapid weight loss, and now you have reached the dreaded plateau. If this becomes the situation for you, you can try a few different strategies:

- Consult your doctor. He may want to run blood tests to rule out any underlying metabolic issues.

- Change up your exercise routine. As the body gets used to any particular form of activity, it becomes more and more efficient at accomplishing the same goals. This means that it gradually burns fewer calories. If you change your exercise routine, you "confuse" your muscles, leading them to work harder and burn more energy again.

- Drink more water. Your body is better at metabolizing energy if it is well hydrated. Just in case you needed one more reason to stay hydrated, there you have it!

- Eat just a little less. Try cutting out one snack, one dessert, or half of a side dish per day to see if just a little more of a deficit helps. Again, you should not take your calorie deficit to extremes!

- Eat just a little more. It is possible your body is too deprived and is beginning to enter into the aforementioned "starvation mode." Many people have discovered that, by eating 200 or so additional healthy calories (lean protein, vegetables, fruit, or whole grains) each day, they were able to meet their weight loss goals.

- Just focus on enjoying your life, healthy nutrition, and surrounding yourself with family and friends. Many people have found that, when they focus on enjoying the positive things of life and stop obsessively counting calories, they can lose weight without much effort gradually.

If you still find yourself plagued by troublesome weight and nothing is working, it may be time to return to your doctor or consult a registered dietician (RD). These professionals can give you the expert guidance you need to troubleshoot your diet and get you pointed in the right direction.

Eating Out on This Diet

Sometimes eating out can be a problem no matter what diet plan or lifestyle you're following. Most items on restaurant menus are filled with salt, fat, and preservatives, making them off-limits.

However, you can still dine out on the Mediterranean diet. Find places to eat that align with your healthy eating habits, such as fresh fruit and vegetable items instead of fried or sauce-laden sides. Also, choose menu items that aren't cooked in butter or heavy sauces, and ask for sauces or dressing to be served on the side so you can control how much you consume.

Many restaurants print the calorie content of their dishes on the menu now, making it easier for us to make health-conscious decisions. If nutritional information is not available on a menu, most chain restaurants have this information listed on their websites. Having this information ahead of time can help you make a smart decision before you even get to the restaurant. That way, you are less likely to fall prey to tempting choices or advertised specials when you arrive at the restaurant.

Ask your server for recommendations, too, or see if he or she could ask the chef to make adjustments for you. You could request a lighter dressing or ask for something to be grilled instead of fried. Remember, you're paying for it, so don't be afraid to ask for what you want politely.

Chapter 6: In Case You're Considering Other Diet

In America, we are often enticed by "quick fix" diets that promise rapid, sustained weight loss. The problem with most of these diets, is that they have no scientific basis, nor is there any long-term data demonstrating their effectiveness regarding steady weight loss or long-term health. Many of these diets can be defined as fad diets, most of which promise that you'll see easy, sudden weight loss. The sad truth is that although some of them may result in initial weight loss, the weight is often quickly gained back. The initial weight loss may not even be healthy weight loss, either. Starving yourself can also lead to weight loss, but it deprives you of the vitamins and nutrients you need to live and can cause permanent damage to your body.

Throughout time, waves of dietary change have come and gone low-fat, nonfat, low-carb, high-carb, vegan, Paleo, etc. These diets are marketed with the promise to promote health and happiness, but they are usually entrenched with all-or-nothing claims, gimmicks, and short-lived dietary plans that are not enjoyable or sustainable. They simply don't (and can't) last.

The Mediterranean diet works. It's easy, and there's no deprivation of any food group. There are recommended *restrictions* of certain foods that aren't beneficial to health, but there are ample choices to maintain variety and satiety for all palettes. Research consistently proves that eating a heart-healthy Mediterranean diet will slash cancer and stroke risks, eradicate preventable diets, and boost the quality of life – not just your quantity of years.

It's no surprise that when following a Mediterranean diet, which promotes healthy fats, produce, whole grains, and seafood, you have lower risks of heart disease and cholesterol, have lower body mass indexes, and experience more heart-healthy benefits. By sticking to healthy portions of fresh food in its natural state, you will obtain all the nutrients needed to nourish the body.

But how can a diet rich in health be healthier than what average Americans eat? Because those fats don't come from animals. Americans consume *saturated* fat, which hinders health. Saturated fats raise cholesterol and can contribute to heart disease. People of the Mediterranean eat *monounsaturated* fat from plant sources, which promotes heart health. Monounsaturated fats help lower levels of cholesterol and reduce our risk of heart disease and stroke. In the famous Seven Countries Study, Ancel Keys observed that the people of Crete, Greece consumed as much as a ½ cup of olive oil per day, per person! He also observed that heart disease rates in the Mediterranean regions of Italy, Spain, and France were incredibly low. It's not always about calories, fat, or protein. It's about the *source* of your food and the *quality* of our ingredients. Despite the substantial scientific evidence behind the Mediterranean diet, you still may be fascinated by one of the many popular diets that have been publicized and popularized in recent years. Here, we'll take a look at some of those diets and discover how the Mediterranean diet stacks up against each one. In some cases, you may be able to find a healthy compromise that combines the Mediterranean diet with another eating plan. In other cases, the Mediterranean way of eating comes out as the clear winner.

The Ketogenic Diet

This is a more trendy diet, recently popularized by social media users, consists of a high-fat, low-carbohydrate, medium-protein eating plan. After you have restricted your consumption of carbohydrates to minimal levels, your metabolism will shift to a process called ketosis, in which your body mobilizes its own carbohydrate stores for fuel because it is not getting enough energy from carbohydrates. The result of this process is thought to be increased burning of the body's fat stores.

With this food pattern, you aim to consume approximately 75% of your calories from fats like avocado, butter, oils, and bacon. Your consumption of fats is almost unlimited, so you get to enjoy some fat-rich choices that most other diets would never allow. You eat about 15 to 20 percent of your calories in protein, which is a moderate amount. Carbohydrate intake is severely limited to only 5 to 10 percent of your diet. This is approximately equivalent to the level of carbohydrates you can find in a couple of apples each day.

By comparison, on the Mediterranean diet, about 50 to 60 percent of your intake is healthy carbohydrates that can be found in fruits, vegetables, and whole grain sources. Fat makes up about a 25 to 35 percent of the diet, with an emphasis on consuming heart-healthy unsaturated fats, found in olive oil, fish, and nuts. Saturated fats, found mainly in animal products, are kept to a minimum.

As you have read throughout this book, the Mediterranean diet is backed by thousands of scientific studies and has been proven to reduce the risk of death from several very svere health issues. On the flip side, the ketogenic diet was initially developed as nutritional therapy for epileptic children! At the time, it was used to help manage seizures in these children. It was never designed for weight loss or the management of other health issues.

The Ketogenic diet is a more challenging and painful way of eating! It limits healthy carbohydrates like whole grains, fruits, and vegetables so severely that it can lead to dangerous deficiencies in essential nutrients. For the sake of your body's natural energy levels, it is challenging, if not impossible, to stick to a low-carb diet for a long time. Additionally, the high levels of saturated fat consumed in the ketogenic diet are dangerous for the health of your cardiovascular system. Eating a lot of animal products rich in saturated fats has been shown to increase your risk of health issues related to circulation and heart health.

Clearly, the winner in this comparison is the Mediterranean diet. It is a safe and healthy solution for long-term weight management and the best chances of enjoying a long, disease-free life. You may be able to lose weight more rapidly with the ketogenic diet, but it is not a wise choice for long-term health or establishing a pattern of wise nutritional decisions.

The Paleo Diet

This diet, which follows the eating patterns of modern man's Stone Age ancestors, is relatively new. Enthusiasts of this diet claim that our bodies were not designed to digest much of what we eat today, and they promote cutting out whole food groups, including grains, dairy, legumes, added sugar, and added salt. The goals of the Paleo diet are the improvement of overall health, weight loss, and decreased risk of diseases.

The Paleo diet has a couple of things in common with the Mediterranean diet. First, both eating plans emphasize the consumption of fresh, whole foods instead of processed foods that contain excessive sugars, salt, and other unhealthy additives. Both diets include nuts, vegetables, fruits, and lean protein sources, all of which have benefits to maintaining a healthy weight, heart health, and lowering the risk of diseases like type 2 diabetes.

However, by cutting out entire food groups, the Paleo diet comes with some risk factors that should be taken into account. Because it excludes dairy, people who follow this diet risk calcium deficiencies. Calcium can be found in leafy greens, but the highest concentration of this critical mineral is in dairy products. Most typical Americans cannot consume the quantity of dark leafy greens required to get their daily recommended amount of calcium. Without enough calcium, we risk developing osteoporosis, numbness in our fingers and toes, convulsions, muscle cramps, and abnormal heart rhythm.

The Paleo diet also cuts out grains and legumes, both of which play essential roles in the Mediterranean diet. Both food groups have been shown to aid digestion, contain vital nutrients, and help prevent serious diseases. Additionally, the Paleo diet can be too high in protein for the average person, which can affect your kidney function.

The bottom line is that the Paleo diet, although not as dangerous as the ketogenic diet, does not stand up to the Mediterranean diet as a well-established and balanced way of eating for long-term health. Additionally, we must consider the fact that significant evolution has taken place in the human digestive system since the Stone Age. Perhaps our ancestors could not have digested grains, legumes, and dairy products. However, now those food groups, in healthy amounts, are easily absorbed by most people and supply important sources of vital nutrients.

Low-Carbohydrate Diets

Both the ketogenic and Paleo diets are forms of low-carbohydrate diets, with the ketogenic diet being a much more extreme version of low-carb eating. Another low-carb diet is the Atkins Diet, which was first publicized more than 30 years ago. This somewhat old fad diet is remarkably similar to the ketogenic diet in that it allows and even encourages the consumption of foods that are high in saturated fat and protein. There is no need to spend much time comparing the Mediterranean diet with the Atkins or other low-carb diets because the basics have already been covered in the last two sections. Depriving the body of essential nutrients found in fruits, vegetables, and whole grains can ultimately be detrimental to health. Replacing carbohydrates with too much fat (especially saturated fat) and protein puts a strain on the kidneys and heart. The Atkins diet and other low-carbohydrate diets may lead to initial rapid weight loss, but studies and anecdotal evidence has shown that this weight loss often slows and sometimes reverses.

Intermittent Fasting

This recent health trend, in contrast with other diets, does not specify what foods to eat and avoid. Instead, it dictates eating patterns in which periods of fasting are alternated with periods of eating.

There are a few patterns of intermittent fasting that are currently popular, and those who wish to try this strategy should take their health, metabolism, gender, activity level, and other lifestyle factors into account when deciding which eating pattern to follow. One pattern is called the 5:2 pattern, in which the dieter normally eats during five days of the week, and drastically restricts his calorie intake for 2 non-consecutive days of each week. Another pattern, the 16/8 method, involves fasting for 16 hours each day and eating normally for only 8 hours a day. A third method is called "eat-stop-eat," and involves fasting for a full 24 hours at a time, once or twice a week.

Intermittent fasting has been shown to help stimulate weight loss because of changes in metabolism and hormone levels that take place when a person enters a fasting phase. Additionally, because all these methods result in the overall reduction of calorie intake, the dieter should lose weight, as long as he does not compensate by eating excessive amounts of food during the "normal eating" periods. Many people find this method easier than other diets because it does not deem any food groups "off-limits." As a result, intermittent fasting can be highly successful in helping you achieve lasting weight loss.

If you do not have any significant health concerns in which fasting causes problems, there is no reason that you should not consider combining the Mediterranean diet with intermittent fasting. Be sure to consult your doctor before embarking on this method, though. He may recommend testing or have some advice about the best fasting and eating pattern for you to follow.

Additionally, if you follow the Mediterranean diet during your eating periods, you will be helping to ensure that your body receives the best nutrition possible during the meals that you do consume. Getting adequate healthy nutrition will help set you up for success in this method, because your body will have received enough fuel to help you make it through the fasting periods.

The DASH and MIND Diets

The DASH, or "Dietary Attempts to Stop Hypertension," diet was initially publicized to help hypertensive patients lower their blood pressure. The Mediterranean diet and the DASH diets have ranked extremely high in recent years as the best eating plans to follow for long-term health.

The two diets are very similar to each other, too. They both encourage the consumption of healthy fats, lean protein sources, whole grains, nuts, legumes, fruits, and vegetables. The critical difference seems to be that the DASH diet allows for more low-fat dairy than the Mediterranean diet.

If you're interested in pursuing both the Mediterranean diet and the DASH diet, there is an easy solution for you. The MIND diet, which is an acronym for the "Mediterranean-DASH Intervention for Neurodegenerative Delay," is a hybrid of these two highly effective diets that aims to reduce the risks of dementia and age-related declines in brain health. The premise behind this diet is that both the Mediterranean and DASH diets have been proven to lower blood pressure, and reduce the risk of several life-threatening diseases. However, neither was created with the goal of improving brain function and preventing dementia. By taking the most brain-healthy elements of both diets, the experts believe they have crafted the best diet for preventing neurodegenerative diseases. The foods recommended on the MIND diet are backed by countless studies and research reviews that show their benefits to brain health.

Rather than focusing on calories or other restrictions, the MIND diet emphasizes the consumption of certain foods over others. Specifically, it recommends that participants eat a lot of green, leafy vegetables along with other vegetables, wine (in moderation, olive oil, fish, berries, poultry, whole grains, and nuts. There are recommended daily, or weekly serving amounts for each of these foods. This diet recommends avoiding butter and margarine, cheese, red meat, fried food, and processed junk food and sweets.

Since the MIND, DASH, and Mediterranean diets are so remarkably similar, you should feel free to try any of the three, depending on your health goals. If you just want a healthy eating plan that helps you enjoy life and reduce your overall risk of disease, the Mediterranean diet is for you. If you have concerns about high blood pressure, you may want to learn more about the DASH diet. If you are focused on protecting your brain health, you should think about following the MIND diet.

The bottom line of this chapter is that it's hard to beat the Mediterranean diet when it comes to an eating plan that promotes long-term health and the enjoyment of life without restricting entire food groups. However, there are variations of this diet that were crafted for people with specific health concerns. If you are one of those people, you can still enjoy the Mediterranean way of life while focusing on your own particular needs.

Chapter 7: Easy Mediterranean Recipes

*NOTE: At the end of each recipe, you'll find a low-carbohydrate variation and a low-sodium variation.

Breakfast Selections

Savory Breakfast Salad

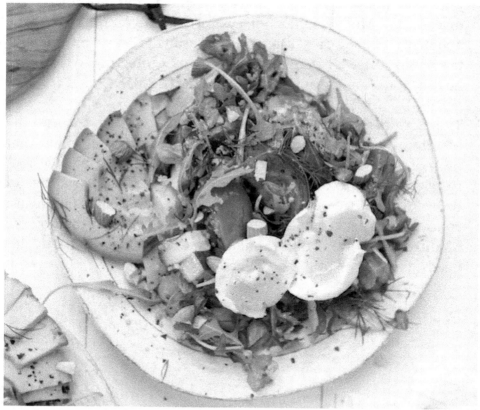

Total Prep and Cooking Time: 15-20 minutes

Nutrition (per serving)
Calories: 519

Fat: 39.4 g.
Carbohydrates: 29.1 g.
Protein: 19.1 g.

Serves 4 people

Although eating a salad for breakfast may seem like a strange idea, so does eating cold leftover pizza from last night – and yet, many of us have woken up on a Saturday morning and eaten a cold slice straight from the fridge. So why not try a healthy option and go for a salad? This dish is loaded with tasty breakfast bites like soft-boiled eggs, tomato, and avocado. Peppery arugula is a delicious non-bread option for soaking up the runny yolks. The healthy fat from avocado and olive oil will help you feel full and energetic until lunch time. To top it off, crunchy almonds and fiber-laden quinoa add even more protein and flavor! Salad for breakfast? Yes, please!

Component
4 eggs, large
2 c. cherry tomatoes, cut in half; or chopped heirloom or Roma tomatoes
10 c. arugula rinsed and patted dry
½ of a seedless cucumber, roughly chopped
1 c. cooked and cooled quinoa
1 c. almonds, chopped (optional: toast the almonds for a flavor boost)
1 large avocado, sliced
½ c. mixed green herbs (examples: mint, dill, or basil)
1 lemon
Salt and pepper
2 Tbsp. extra-virgin olive oil, for drizzling

Preparation:

1. Soft-boil the eggs. Heat a pot of cold water until it boils, then lower the heat until the liquid is simmering (gently bubbling, or just below boiling). Then gently place the eggs in the water with a large spoon and leave them in the simmering water for 6 minutes. Remove them promptly from the pot and run them under cold water immediately. Set the eggs aside; peel them when you are ready to use them.

2. Place the following ingredients in a large bowl: chopped tomatoes, chopped cucumber, cold cooked quinoa, and arugula. Toss to combine, then drizzle about half of the oil over it. Season with the ground pepper and salt, then toss again.

3. Divide the mixture from the bowl between four plates. Next, peel the eggs and cut them in half. Soon after, top each salad with one-halved egg and ¼ of the sliced avocado. Sprinkle the mixed herbs and almonds evenly over the top of the four salads. Top each salad by gently squeezing a little lemon juice over it, sprinkling a bit more salt and pepper (to taste), and drizzling the rest of the olive oil over it. Share and enjoy!

Low-Carbohydrate Variation: Cut the number of vegetables in half and eliminate the quinoa. Add one more egg per person and double the almonds.

Low-Sodium Variation: Do not use any salt.

Almond-Honey Ricotta and Peaches on English Muffin

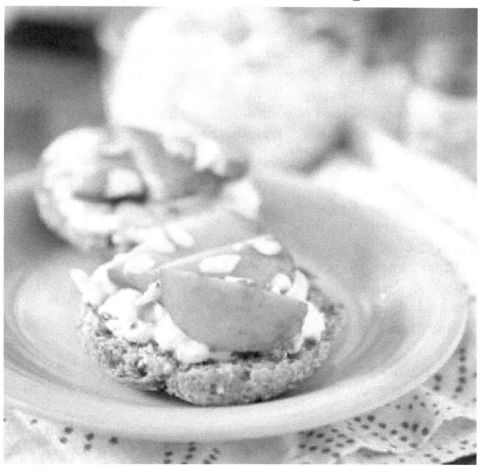

Total Prep and Cooking Time: 10 minutes

<u>Nutrition (per serving)</u>
Calories: 391
Fat: 17.4 g.
Carbohydrates: 46.8 g.
Protein: 16.6 g.

Serves 4 people

In contrast to some more savory breakfast dishes, this dish will satisfy anyone who wakes up with a craving for something sweet. The almonds and whole-wheat muffin, in addition to the fat from ricotta cheese, help give you sustainable energy. Peaches and honey add healthy sources of sweetness and vital nutrients to the start of your day. If you like to begin with a stack of syrupy pancakes, try this meal out for a healthy Mediterranean substitute.

Components

4 whole-grain English muffins
1 c. whole milk ricotta
5 tsp honey
¼ tsp almond extract
½ c. sliced almonds
2 medium ripe peaches, pitted and sliced
orange zest (optional)

Preparation

1. Separate the halves of the English muffins and toast them.
2. While the muffins are toasting, combine the following items in a small bowl: Ricotta cheese, 1 tsp. of the honey, almonds (set aside a few for sprinkling over the tops, if you like), almond extract, and orange zest (almonds). Stir it all together gently.
3. Spread approximately 1/8 of the mixture over each muffin half. Top with the peach slices, extra almonds that you set aside, and about ½ tsp. of honey per muffin half. Share and enjoy!

Low-Carbohydrate Variation: Serve the spread wrapped in a low-carb wrap. Use one peach instead of two. Add more almonds for increased satiety.

Avocado, Smoked Salmon, and Poached Eggs on Toast

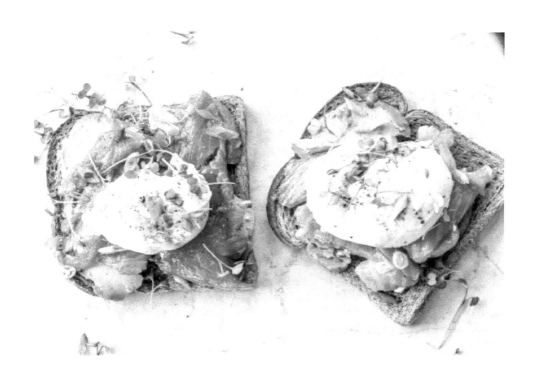

Total Prep and Cooking Time: 15-20 minutes

Nutrition (per serving)
Calories: 463
Fat: 22.4 g.
Carbohydrates: 30.2 g.
Protein: 35.0 g.

Serves 1 person

When it comes to protein-packed breakfasts, this one carries the motherlode! Thanks to savory smoked salmon and two eggs, you'll definitely be satisfied by this tasty beginning to your day. Add the creamy deliciousness of avocado and sharp peppery arugula, and your taste buds will be in heaven. While the smoked salmon is slightly less budget-friendly than most of the ingredients in this book, it is well worth the occasional splurge. This dish has everything you need for a satisfying start to a productive weekday, or a weekend brunch so tasty you can scarcely believe it's good for you.

Components

2 slices whole grain bread, toasted
¼ large avocado
lemon juice, just a few drops
2 large eggs
¼ c. arugula
3 oz. smoked salmon
salt and pepper, if desired

Preparation

1. Within a small bowl, mash up ¼ avocado thoroughly. Add the lemon juice, a tiny sprinkle of salt, stir and set this dish aside.
2. Poach the eggs, one at a time. See the instructions below if you've never poached an egg.
3. Divide the avocado mash in half and spread it over both slices of bread. Adorn the mashed avocado with the arugula leaves, then add ½ of the smoked salmon to each slice.
4. Gently place a poached egg on top of each slice, then sprinkle with salt and pepper to your liking.

5. Even though this meal is served on toast, you'll need a fork and knife to eat it!

Egg Poaching Directions:
1. Always poach eggs one at a time.
2. Heat a small pot of water until it is simmering (gently bubbling or almost boiling).
3. Crack the eggs cleanly into individual small bowls.
4. Use a large spoon to stir the simmering water until it moves smoothly in a circle, like a whirlpool.
5. Softly tip one egg into the swirling water and leave it in there for two minutes.
6. Remove the egg gently with a slotted spoon and put it in ice water for just about 10 seconds to stop the cooking process (this will keep the yolk runny).
7. Use a paper towel to pat the egg dry and use the edge of a spoon to cut off any wispy whites from around the egg.

Low-Carbohydrate Variation: Eliminate the bread and serve the other ingredients in a bowl. Double the avocado and consider adding more smoked salmon.

Low-Sodium Variation: Use fresh salmon that has been grilled, broiled, or poached instead of smoked salmon.

Berry Good Greek Yogurt Pancakes

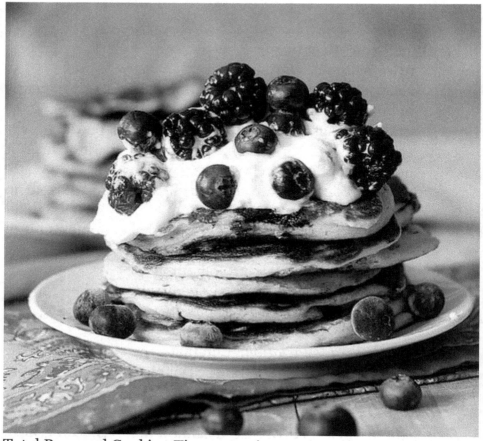

Total Prep and Cooking Time: 30 minutes

<u>Nutrition (per serving)</u>
Calories: 301
Fat: 9.4 g.
Carbohydrates: 37.9 g.
Protein: 19.0 g.

Serves 6 people

Even though pancakes seem like a decadent treat that you shouldn't touch with a ten-foot pole when you're following a healthy eating plan, there actually is a way to enjoy them on the Mediterranean Diet! When you use whole wheat flour, limit the sugar, skip the syrup on top, and add protein-packed Greek yogurt to the mix, even pancakes can be relatively healthy! Topped with yummy berries, this family-friendly recipe is sure to be a crowd pleaser.

Components

1 ¼ c. flour (preferably whole-wheat)
2 tsp. baking powder
1 tsp. of baking soda
¼ c. of sugar
¼ tsp. salt
3 c. nonfat plain Greek yogurt, divided in half
3 T. extra virgin olive oil
½ c. nonfat (skim) milk
1 ½ c. blueberries or other berries of your choosing

Preparation

1. Within a mixing bowl, add all the following ingredients: flour, salt, and baking powder and soda. Combine them all together with a whisk.
2. Within a different bowl, add the oil, sugar, 1 ½ c. of the yogurt, and the milk. Use a whisk to blend them until smooth vigorously.
3. Gently combine the two mixtures (from step 1 and step 2) together. Use a spoon to form a smooth batter. For one option, gently stir in the berries. Otherwise, leave them out and use them for a topping when serving.
4. Warm a skillet or pancake griddle. Test by sprinkling water on the hot surface – if the water droplets sizzle on

the surface, it's ready. Spray the hot surface with non-stick oil spray.

5. Pour the batter, ¼ c. at a time, onto the cooking surface. When bubbles on the wet surface pop and leave small holes, check the bottom edges to see if it's golden brown, then flip the pancake (use a wide spatula).

6. Place pancakes on a plate in a warm oven until ready to serve.

7. Serve topped with the remainder of the Greek yogurt and the berries (unless you incorporated them into the batter). Delicious!

Low-Carbohydrate Variation: The central part of this meal is carbohydrates, so you may want to avoid this dish altogether if you're cutting carbs. Instead, enjoy a bowl of Greek yogurt with a few blueberries.

Low-Sodium Variation: Eliminate the salt from the recipe.

Veggie Egg Cups with Feta

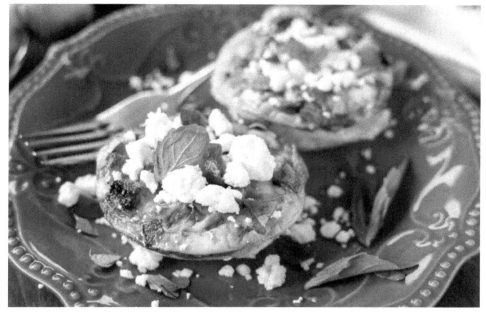

Total Prep and Cooking Time: 35-45 minutes

<u>Nutrition (per two egg cups)</u>
Calories: 229
Fat: 17 grams
Carbohydrates: 4.6 grams
Protein: 15.3 grams

Serves 6 people

If you're a fan of preparing food a day or so before you need it, you'll love these delightful little egg cups! You can make them the night before and warm them up the next morning, or even serve them cold if you're in a hurry. The recipe serves six people, but we won't tell anyone if you eat it all yourself, spread out over six different mornings! If you're following a low-carb Mediterranean diet hybrid plan, this dish requires no modifications, as it barely contains any carbohydrates, to begin with. This version includes roasted red peppers and mushrooms, but you can feel free to substitute any other vegetable you have on hand.

Components
10 large eggs
nonstick cooking spray
2/3 c. of nonfat (skim) milk
½ tsp. garlic powder
1/8 tsp. of salt
¼ tsp. ground pepper
1 ½ c. raw mushrooms, cleaned and chopped
1 ½ cup roasted red peppers, drained, rinsed, and dried
1 c. feta cheese
fresh basil leaves, for garnish

Preparation
1. Warm up your oven until it reaches 350 degrees (F). You'll need a muffin tin with 12 cups that has been prepared with cooking spray.
2. Break all the eggs into a bowl, then add the milk, garlic powder, salt, and black pepper. Use a whisk to combine them all. Then add the mushrooms and peppers and stir until the vegetables are uniformly distributed.
3. Using a ladle, distribute the mixture evenly into the 12 cups of the muffin tin. It's okay if the cups are quite full.
4. Place muffin tin in the oven and leave for 25 minutes, or whenever the eggs look completely set (not runny or jiggly when the pan is shaken lightly).
5. Leave egg cups in the muffin tin to cool for 5 to 10 minutes. They will appear to deflate a little. Then remove them from the tin.

6. Serve 2 egg cups per serving. Top with feta cheese (divided into 6 portions) and basil leaves.

7.

Low-Carbohydrate Variation: This is a low-carb recipe without any changes necessary.

Low-Sodium Variation: Eliminate the salt in the recipe and sprinkle part-skim mozzarella on the egg cups instead of feta cheese.

Lunch Selections

Chickpea Lettuce Wraps

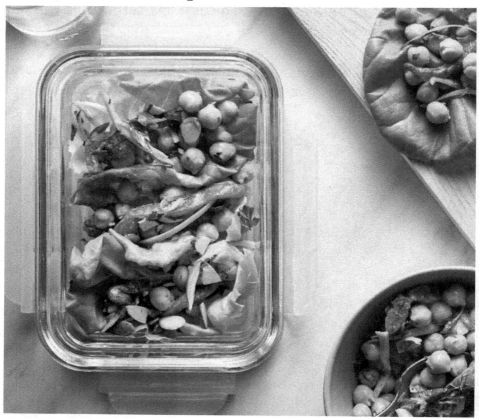

Total Prep and Cooking Time: 10 minutes

<u>Nutrition (per serving)</u>
Calories: 516
Fat: 32.3 g.
Carbohydrates: 46.1 g.
Protein: 17.3 g.

Serves 4 people

This tasty lunch option easy to prepare ahead of time and bring to work, or you can make it at home for a light to share with family or friends. It's chock-full of the trademark Mediterranean flavors and nutrients, and it's guaranteed to satisfy. Although it's high in carbohydrates, you must keep in mind that these are *healthy* carbohydrates, from vegetables and legumes. Your body will take its time breaking down the tasty, fiber-filled little chickpeas, and your taste buds will thank you for the flavor of the tangy tahini dressing and the crunch of toasted almonds in this no-cook, easy-to-prepare meal.

Components
¼ c. tahini (a paste made from ground-up sesame seeds; refrigerate after opening)
¼ c. extra-virgin olive oil
1 teaspoon lemon zest
¼ c. juice from lemons (approximately the juice from 2 lemons)
1 ½ tsp. of pure maple syrup
¾ tsp. salt
½ teaspoon paprika
2 (15 oz.) cans chickpeas (no salt added), drained and rinsed
½ c. of Jarred sliced roasted red bell peppers, drained
½ c. thinly sliced shallots or green onions
12 large lettuce leaves – Bibb, butter, or Romaine are recommended, but any type that makes a good wrap will do
¼ c. chopped toasted almonds
2 Tbsp. parsley, fresh and minced

Preparation
1. Place the sheet of meatballs on the middle rack of the heated oven and bake them 20-22 minutes. They should be golden brown before you take them out of the oven. Allow them to cool off outside the oven.

2. While the meatballs bake, make the yogurt dip. Add all the components of the sauce to a small bowl and whisk them together until thoroughly combined. Cover the bowl and chill until ready to serve.
3. Keep meatballs and yogurt in the refrigerator until ready to serve. The meatballs will keep for 3 to 4 days, and the dip will keep for 7 to 10 days.
4. Enjoy!

Low-Carbohydrate Variation: This is a low-carb recipe. You can use more lentils and fewer breadcrumbs if you like, but this may change the texture too much.

Low-Sodium Variation: Eliminate the table salt. Use mozzarella instead of feta cheese.

Quinoa Chicken Power Bowl

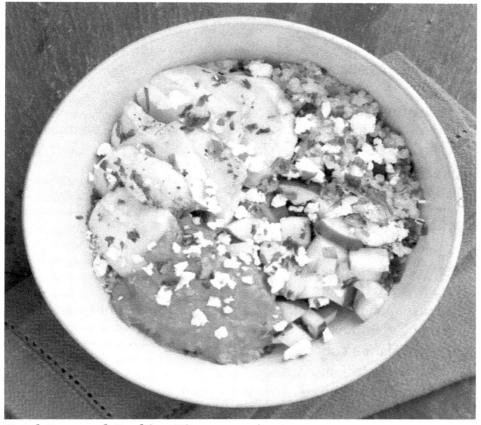

Total Prep and Cooking Time: 30 minutes

Nutrition (per serving)
Calories: 520
Fat: 27 g.
Carbohydrates: 31 g.
Protein: 34 g.

Serves 4 people

Fresh ingredients seem to come together magically in this well-balanced, nutritious dish. This is another lunch that travels well and can be prepared in advance. Just cook the components ahead of time, bring them to work, and assemble the parts just before eating. You'll be wowed by how delicious a protein-packed power bowl can be when you taste the spices that blend easily into a delicious sauce.

Components

1 pound of chicken breasts (boneless and skinless), trimmed
¼ tsp. of salt
¼ tsp. black pepper
1 (7 oz.) jar red peppers, rinsed
¼ c. slivered almonds
4 T. extra-virgin olive oil
1 clove of crushed garlic
1 teaspoon paprika
½ tsp. ground cumin
¼ teaspoon crushed red pepper flakes (optional for extra spice)
2 c. cooked quinoa
¼ cup Kalamata olives, diced
¼ cup red onion, minced
1 c. of cucumber, diced
¼ c. crumbled Feta cheese
2 Tbsp. fresh parsley, minced

Preparation

1. Turn on oven broiler at "high" setting, with the rack in the upper third of the oven. Place foil over the top of a baking sheet.
2. Sprinkle the pepper and salt on the chicken breasts and put them on the foil-covered baking sheet. Broil the chicken for 14 to 18 minutes, turning over halfway through the time. They are cooked when the internal temperature (read with a meat thermometer) reads 165 degrees Fahrenheit.

3. Use a sharp knife or forks to slice or shred the cooked chicken breasts on a cutting board.
4. While the chicken cooks, add the following components to a small food processor: half of the oil (2 tablespoons), peppers, garlic, almonds, cumin, paprika, and crushed red pepper flakes (optional). Puree all of these together until they form a relatively smooth sauce.
5. In a medium bowl, add the following components: quinoa, the rest of the olive oil (2 tablespoons), red onion, and olives. Use a large spoon to stir them together.
6. Serve by dividing the quinoa mixture between 4 bowls. Top each bowl with equal amounts of the chicken, cucumber, and red pepper sauce. Over the top, sprinkle parsley and feta cheese.
7. If making this dish ahead of time, store the chicken, sauce, and quinoa mixture in three separate containers and combine just before serving.
8. One serving is 3 oz. of chicken, ¼ c. of the sauce, and ½ c. of the quinoa.
9. Enjoy!

Low-Carbohydrate Variation: Use 1 cup of quinoa and 1 ½ pound of chicken.

Low-Sodium Variation: Take out the table salt, eliminate the kalamata olives, and substitute part-skim mozzarella cheese for feta cheese.

Tuscany Tuna Salad in Pita

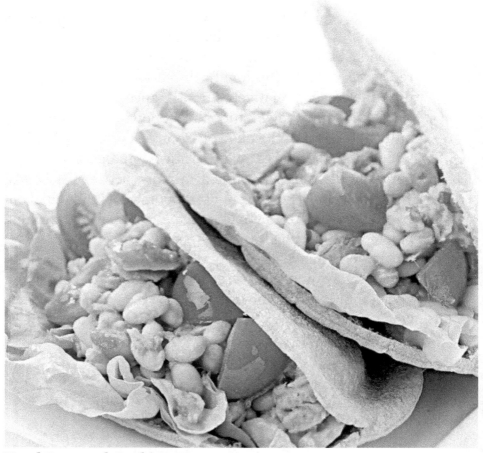

Total Prep and Cooking Time: 10 minutes

Nutrition (per serving)
Calories: 322
Fat: 9.8 g.
Carbohydrates: 45.1 g.
Protein: 20.7 g.

Serves 4 people

This meal represents a simplified version of a northern Italian dish. It's quick and easy to prepare and can be stored in the refrigerator for a few days. This light but filling fare is also versatile – serve it in a bowl, in a wrap, on a sandwich, or in a pita pocket as this recipe instructs. It's perfect for lunch in the office or a warm summer evening on the porch. The suggested tuna for this salad is chunk light, packed in water, because it is lower in mercury than white albacore tuna and lower in fat than tuna packed in oil.

Components
2 small cans drained chunk light tuna
4 green onions (scallions), sliced
10 cherry tomatoes, washed and quartered
2 Tbsp. extra virgin olive oil
2 Tbsp. lemon juice
¼ tsp. salt
1 (15 oz.) can of drained and rinsed cannellini beans
ground black pepper, to taste
lettuce leaves, any variety of your choosing
4 pieces of medium pita bread (5 ¼ inch diameter), with pockets inside

Preparation:
1. Add the following ingredients to a medium bowl: tomatoes, tuna, beans, olive oil, green onions, lemon juice, pepper, and salt. Use a spoon to stir it all together gently. Cover and refrigerate the salad until ready to serve.
2. To serve, line the inside of the pita bread pockets with lettuce and scoop one cup of the tuna salad on top of the lettuce. Enjoy!

Low-Carbohydrate Variation: Serve the tuna salad in a lettuce wrap instead of a pita pocket.

Low-Sodium Variation: Eliminate the table salt and use "very low sodium" canned white albacore tuna in water instead of chunk light tuna. The white albacore tuna, however, has more mercury, so it is not advisable for pregnant women and for children.

Beet and Shrimp Salad

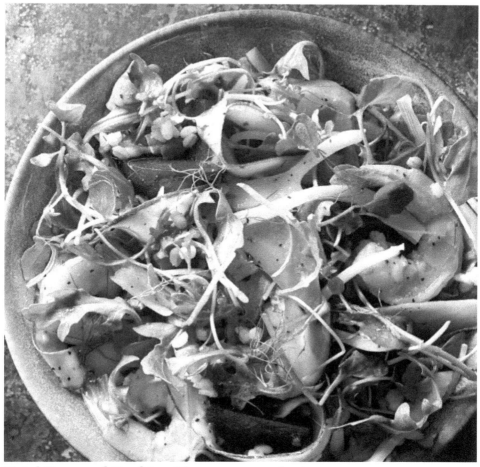

Total Prep and Cooking Time: 15-20 minutes

Nutrition (per serving)
Calories: 584
Fat: 30 g.
Carbohydrates: 47 g.
Protein: 35 g.

Serves 1 person

At first glance, the amount of fat in this mouth-watering salad may frighten you, but of the 30 grams of fat, only 4 grams is saturated fat! That means that the rest is heart-healthy, appetite-satisfying monounsaturated or polyunsaturated fat. Packed with tasty and nutritious veggies and fiber-full barley, this Beet and Shrimp Salad will brighten up the dreariest day and give you an energy boost that you need to get through your afternoon. This recipe only serves one, but it can easily be doubled, tripled, or even quadrupled when you're serving friends or family.

Components

2 c. arugula

1 c. watercress

1 c. cooked beet wedges (usually found with other prepared vegetables in your   grocery store's produce   department)

½ c. zucchini ribbons (see step 1 for preparation)

½ c. of thinly sliced fennel

½ c. cooked barley

4 oz. cooked, peeled shrimp (fresh or frozen and thawed)

2 Tbsp. extra-virgin olive oil

1 Tbsp. wine vinegar (red or white, your preference)

½ tsp. mustard (preferably Dijon)

½ teaspoon minced shallot

¼ teaspoon ground pepper

1/8 teaspoon salt

Preparation

1. To make zucchini ribbons, use a vegetable peeler to shave a whole zucchini lengthwise thinly.
2. On a plate, arrange the watercress, beet wedges, arugula, zucchini ribbons, fennel, shrimp, and barley.
3. Add the following ingredients to a small bowl or bottle: salt, pepper, mustard, minced shallot, olive oil, and wine

vinegar. Combine with a whisk in a bowl or shake in a closed bottle until thoroughly mixed.

4. Drizzle dressing over the salad and enjoy!

Low-Carbohydrate Variation: Use half the beets, eliminate the barley, and use 6 ounces of shrimp.

Low-Sodium Variation: Eliminate the table salt.

Italian Veggie Sandwich

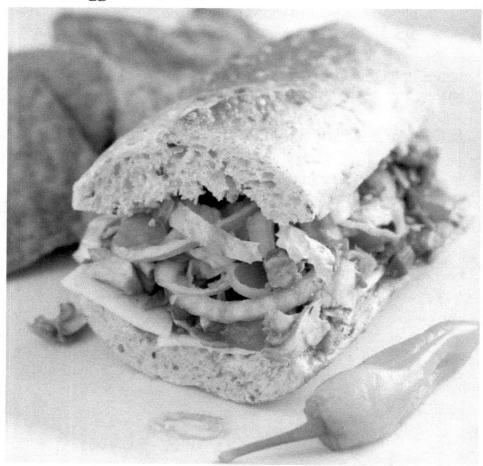

Total Prep and Cooking Time: 20 minutes

Nutrition (per serving)
Calories: 266
Fat: 8 g.
Carbohydrates: 40 g.
Protein: 14 g.

Serves 4 people

These sub-style sandwiches are a little messy but delightfully zesty and full of fun textures and flavors. They're great for serving at home, on a picnic, or bringing for lunch at the office. One suggestion is to pack the bread and other components separately, then assemble them right before eating. This way, you'll avoid soggy bread! Serve with a salad for even more veggies in your meal.

Components

¼ c. red onion, thinly sliced, rings separated
1 can of artichoke hearts, rinsed, sliced
1 Roma tomato, diced
1 Tbsp. extra-virgin olive oil
2 Tbsp. balsamic vinegar
1 teaspoon oregano
1 baguette, approximately 20" long, whole grain if possible
2 slices provolone cheese, cut in half
2 c. of romaine lettuce, shredded
¼ c. pepperoncini (optional, for spice)

Preparation:

1. Place onion rings in a bowl of cold water and set aside while you make the rest of the sandwich.
2. In a medium bowl, place the following components: tomato, artichoke hearts, oregano, oil, vinegar.
3. Cut the baguette into four equivalent portions, then divide them horizontally. Pull out about half the insides from the pieces of bread.
4. Drain the onions from the water and pat dry.
5. For sandwich assembly: place one half-slice of cheese on the bottom half of a baguette portion, then cover with ¼ of the tomato-artichoke mixture. Place ¼ of the lettuce and pepperoncini on top, then place the top half of the baguette upon the sandwich.

6. Serve right away after assembling. Enjoy!

Low-Carbohydrate Variation: Serve ingredients in a lettuce wrap or a low-carbohydrate wrap instead of on a baguette.

Low-Sodium Variation: Rinse the artichoke hearts thoroughly to eliminate any added salt from the canning juices. Use sliced mozzarella cheese instead of provolone. Do not use the pepperoncini peppers.

Dinner Selections

Tomato and Ricotta Whole-Grain Pasta

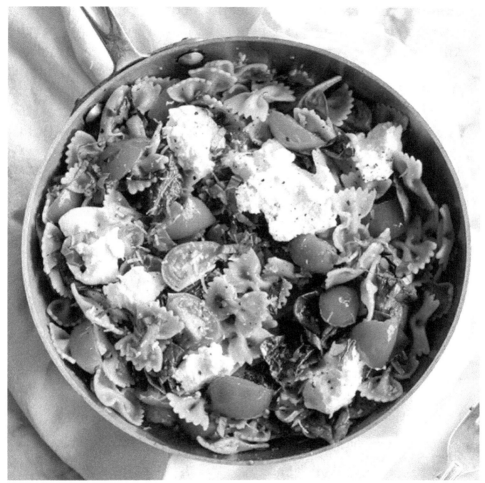

Total Prep and Cooking Time: 25 minutes

Nutrition (per serving)
Calories: 519
Fat: 29.9 g.
Carbohydrates: 48 g.
Protein: 21.6 g.

Serves 4 people

Although the Mediterranean diet does not contain a whole lot of the carb-heavy pasta most people associate with Italy, there is still a place for whole-grain noodles, eaten in moderation and served with plenty of vegetables! This nutritious dish contains plenty of protein and calcium from ricotta cheese, along with fiber from the whole-wheat pasta. Bright, healthy tomatoes and spinach round out the meal for a flavorful main course that's sure to be a crowd-pleaser. Best of all, it's quick and easy to make.

Components

8 oz. whole-wheat short pasta (like elbow macaroni, medium shells, or farfalle)
1/3 cup extra-virgin olive oil
3 cloves of garlic, finely minced
8 to 10 cocktail-sized tomatoes, cut into quarters
salt and ground pepper, as much as desired
2 c. fresh leaves of spinach
1/3 c. fresh basil, sliced
½ cup parmesan cheese, grated
1 cup of ricotta cheese

Preparation:

1. Cook pasta in boiling water for about 1 minute less than package instructions, so pasta is "al dente." Drain, but first set aside ¼ c. of pasta water.
2. Place a large frying pan or sautéing pan on a stove burner. Set to medium and warm up the oil in it. Add the garlic, then set the heat down a little lower. Stir and cook the garlic for five minutes, watching to be sure it doesn't burn, then add the tomatoes. Sprinkle on pepper and salt

as desired. Cook an additional 2-3 minutes until tomatoes are warm.

3. In the pan with the tomatoes and garlic, add the cooked pasta and spinach. Use tongs or a large spoon to toss until the spinach starts wilting gently. Then include the basil, parmesan cheese, and more salt and pepper if desired. Add a little of the pasta water (1-2 tablespoons) or more olive oil if the pasta seems dry at this point.

4. Top the pasta off by dropping scoops of the ricotta cheese on top and serve. Enjoy!

Low-Carbohydrate Variation: Use low-carbohydrate pasta. Alternatively, cook and prepare all the ingredients except the pasta. Serve over boneless, skinless chicken breast or fish.

Low-Sodium Variation: Use low-sodium pasta.

Spiced Salmon with Vegetable Quinoa

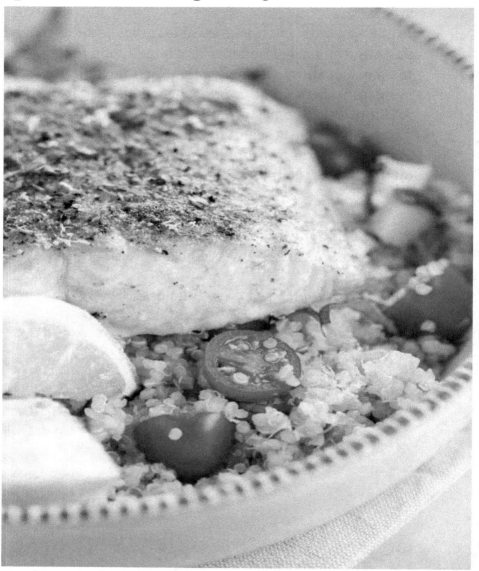

Total Prep and Cooking Time: 30 minutes

Nutrition (per serving)
Calories: 385
Fat: 12.5 g.

Carbohydrates: 32.5 g.
Protein: 35.5 g.

Serves 4 people

This dish looks so fancy you'd expect it could be served at a restaurant, but the truth is that you can whip it up in just a half hour. The salmon is perfectly seasoned for a combination of heat and pure flavor, and the quinoa is livened up with bright vegetables. The best part is that this dish packs a punch of a whopping 35 grams of protein! What a way to finish off your day.

Components
1 c. uncooked quinoa
1 tsp. of salt, divided in half
¾ c. cucumbers, seeds removed, diced
1 c. of cherry tomatoes, halved
¼ c. red onion, minced
4 fresh basil leaves, cut in thin slices
zest from one lemon
¼ teaspoon black pepper
1 teaspoon cumin
½ teaspoon paprika
4 (5-oz.) salmon fillets
8 lemon wedges
¼ c. fresh parsley, chopped

Preparation:
1. To a medium-sized saucepan, add the quinoa, 2 cups of water, and ½ tsp. of the salt. Heat these until the water is boiling, then lower the temperature until it is simmering. Cover the pan and let it cook 20 minutes or as long as the quinoa package instructs.

2. Turn off the burner under the quinoa and allow it to sit, covered, for at least another 5 minutes before serving.
3. Right before serving, add the onion, tomatoes, cucumbers, basil leaves, and lemon zest to the quinoa and use a spoon to stir everything together gently.
4. In the meantime (while the quinoa cooks), prepare the salmon. Turn on the oven broiler to high and make sure a rack is in the lower part of the oven.
5. To a small bowl, add the following components: black pepper, ½ tsp. of the salt, cumin, and paprika. Stir them together.
6. Place foil over the top of a glass or aluminum baking sheet, then spray it with nonstick cooking spray.
7. Place salmon fillets on the foil. Rub the spice mixture over the surface of each fillet (about ½ tsp. of the spice mixture per fillet).
8. Add the lemon wedges to the pan edges near the salmon.
9. Cook the salmon under the broiler for 8-10 minutes. Your goal is for the salmon to flake apart easily with a fork.
10. Sprinkle the salmon with the parsley, then serve it with the lemon wedges and vegetable parsley. Enjoy!
11.

Low-Carbohydrate Variation: Substitute wilted spinach leaves for half the quinoa. Increase the size of the salmon fillets, if desired.

Low-Sodium Variation: Eliminate the table salt.

Easy Lamb Kofta with Chickpeas and Naan

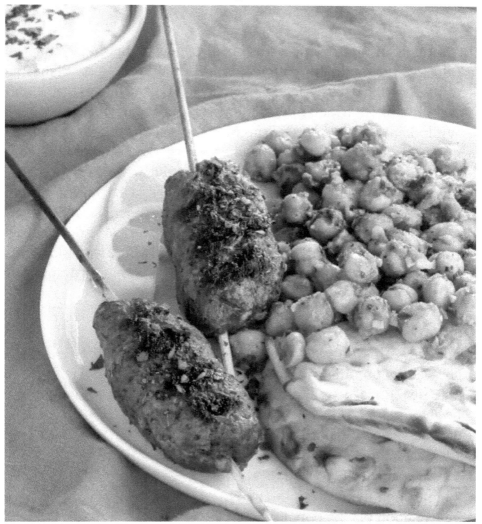

Total Prep and Cooking Time: 60 minutes

Nutrition (per serving)

Calories: 601
Fat: 38 g.
Carbohydrates: 38 g.
Protein: 30 g.

Serves 4 people

Although at first glance this meal seems a bit heavy on the calories, the numbers you see above include the side dishes as well. This meal is perfectly balanced between fat, protein, and carbohydrates, which makes it entirely satisfying and nutritious. While healthy followers of the Mediterranean diet don't eat red meat very often, there is indeed room for the occasional Greek-style lamb *kofta* (meatball) kebobs! Served with a fresh yogurt sauce, a simple side of sautéed chickpeas with harissa paste (easily found in the ethnic section of most grocery stores), and a small portion of naan (Indian flatbread), this meal is deceptively simple to make. Your guests or family will think you slaved in the kitchen for hours, but you'll know it was a matter of an hour or less.

Components
For the kofta
3 T. red onion, finely minced
3 T. mixed fresh Italian herbs (like parsley, mint, and cilantro), finely minced
3 minced cloves of garlic
1 ¼ teaspoon salt
1 teaspoon cumin
¾ teaspoon paprika
½ teaspoon black pepper
1 lb. ground lamb (ask for the lean ground lamb to minimize saturated fat; can substitute lean ground beef)
nonstick cooking spray
skewers for cooking the meat

For the sauce
½ c. plain nonfat yogurt

1 tsp. mixed fresh Italian herbs, finely minced
2 tsp. fresh lemon juice
pinch of salt

For the chickpeas
4 Tbsp. extra-virgin olive oil, divided in half
1 T. red onion, minced
1 garlic clove, minced
1 can chickpeas, rinsed and drained
1 tsp. harissa paste (North African hot sauce, found in Mediterranean section of grocery stores)
¾ tsp. of ground cumin
½ tsp. of paprika
salt, to taste
¼ c. low-sodium chicken stock
1 teaspoon lemon juice
1 T. mixed fresh Italian herbs, finely minced

For serving
1 store-bought flatbread or naan, preferably whole-wheat, divided into 4 pieces

Preparation:
*Note: You'll notice that the chickpeas, sauce, and kofta all have the same Italian herbs in them. You can save time by chopping all the herbs together ahead of time, instead of individually for each dish.

1. *Prepare the kofta meat:* In a stand mixer's bowl, add all the kofta components except the meat itself. Mix on slow speed with a beater blade until these parts are combined. Then incorporate the meat by beating until thoroughly combined with the other parts. Use plastic wrap to cover this bowl and refrigerate it until ready to cook the meat. Meanwhile, prepare the rest of the dishes.

2. When ready to cook the meat, grab a handful and form it into an oblong, sausage-like shape (see picture), then stick a skewer through it. You can also make any other shape you like with the meat – patties, meatballs, etc.- and you do not have to use skewers.

3. Set a large pan or griddle on med-high heat and spray it generously with nonstick cooking spray. When the surface is very hot, cook the meat skewers for 3 to 4 minutes per side, until deep golden on both sides and cooked thoroughly.

4. *Make the yogurt sauce:* Within a bowl, place yogurt, herbs, lemon juice, and salt. Use a whisk or spoon to stir thoroughly and set aside.

5. *Cook the chickpeas:* Set a large sautéing pan on the stove over a burner set to medium. Heat up 2 Tbsp. of the oil, then cook the onions in the heated oil for one to two minutes, until they become just softened. Then incorporate the garlic and sauté for another thirty seconds.

6. Next, add the harissa, chickpeas, paprika, cumin, salt, and chicken stock. Increase the heat under the pan to high and cook while stirring until almost all the stock has evaporated.

7. Remove pan from heat and add the lemon juice and herbs, then stir. Add the rest of the oil right before you serve it.

8. *To serve:* Divide meatballs and chickpeas among 4 plates. Add a ¼ piece of naan or whole-wheat flatbread to each

plate. Serve with yogurt sauce for dipping or drizzling over meatballs. Enjoy!

Low-Carbohydrate Variation: Serve a salad or sautéed vegetables instead of chickpeas. Eliminate the flatbread.

Low-Sodium Variation: Eliminate the table salt. Use unsalted chicken broth instead of low-sodium chicken broth.

Slow-Cooker Mediterranean Chicken with Quinoa

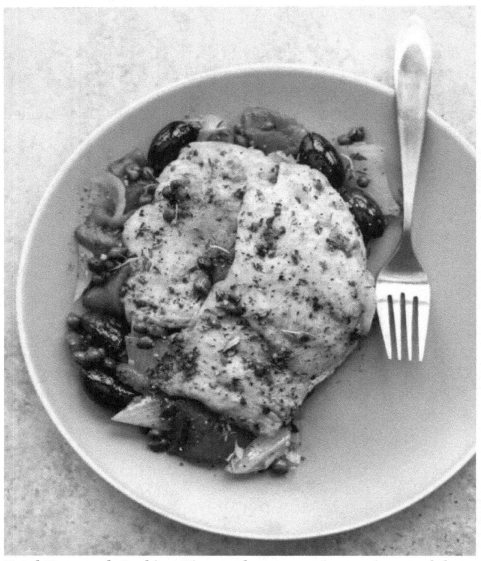

Total Prep and Cooking Time: 4 hours, 5 minutes (most of the time is inactive, while chicken cooks in the slow cooker)

<u>Nutrition (per serving; with quinoa)</u>
Calories: 356
Fat: 11 grams

Carbohydrates: 35 grams
Protein: 30.2 grams

Nutrition (per serving; without quinoa)
Calories: 200
Fat: 8.6 g.
Carbohydrates: 7.6 g.
Protein: 24.2 g.

Serves 4 people

You've got to love the slow cooker concept – start a meal in the morning or the middle of the day, go about your business, and voila! You have dinner when you come home later. The convenience of this kitchen gadget cannot be overstated, not to mention the joy of coming home to the wonderful smells of dinner already cooking. This simple but delicious dish combines classic Mediterranean flavors with the lean protein of boneless, skinless chicken breasts. Serve it with some quinoa, and you've got a complete meal! This is an easy dish that will quickly become a family favorite.

Components:
nonstick cooking spray
4 medium chicken breasts (boneless and skinless; about 4 oz. each)
salt and pepper, as much as desired
3 tsp. Italian seasoning
2 Tbsp. lemon juice
1 Tbsp. garlic, minced
1 medium onion, roughly chopped
1 c. kalamata olives
1 c. jarred red peppers, drained, diced
2 T. capers

fresh basil or thyme for garnish (optional)
1 cup uncooked quinoa

Preparation:

1. Sprinkle pepper and salt over the chicken breasts. Warm a skillet on stove burner over med-low heat and cook chicken for one or two minutes on each side, or just until becoming brown.
2. Spray inside the slow cooker with nonstick spray and put in the browned chicken breasts. Add olives, capers, red peppers, and onion around the sides of the breasts, not over the top.
3. Within a bowl, place the following components: lemon juice, Italian seasoning, and garlic. Use a whisk to combine them. Pour this mixture over the components of the slow cooker.
4. Cover the slow cooker; cook on low heat for 4 hours. You can also cook it on high for 2 hours.
5. When it is almost time for dinner, cook the quinoa according to package directions.
6. To serve, divide the quinoa among 4 plates, then top with one chicken breast on each plate. Divide the rest of the crockpot ingredients between the 4 plates and serve. Enjoy!

Low-Carbohydrate Variation: Serve on a bed of greens instead of quinoa. Use more chicken if desired.

Low-Sodium Variation: Eliminate the table salt and kalamata olives.

Speedy Shrimp Puttanesca

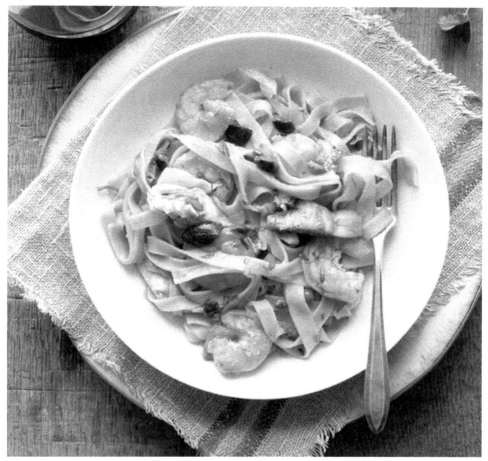

Total Prep and Cooking Time: 15 minutes

<u>Nutrition (per serving)</u>
Calories: 390
Fat: 8 g.
Carbohydrates: 43 g.
Protein: 37 g.

Serves 4 people

Fresh pasta (found in the refrigerated section of your grocery store) cooks much faster than dried pasta so the dish can be on your table swiftly! Puttanesca is usually made with anchovies, capers, olives, tomatoes, and garlic; however, here it gets a protein boost from the shrimp and a fiber boost from artichokes. You'll love the flavor combination and the ease with which you can prepare this meal for yourself and your family.

Components

8 oz. fresh refrigerated linguini noodles, whole-wheat if possible

1 T. extra-virgin olive oil

1 pound peeled, deveined large shrimp (fresh or frozen and thawed)

1 medium can of tomato sauce, without added salt

1 ¼ c. artichoke hearts, quartered (purchase frozen or canned; drain if canned)

¼ c. Kalamata olives, pitted and chopped

1 T. capers, rinsed

¼ tsp. of salt

Preparation:

1. Place a large pot of water on a stove burner set on high and heat until the water is boiling. Cook the linguini as the package instructs, and then drain.

2. Pour the oil in a large sautéing pan and heat it on high. Place shrimp in hot oil in a single layer. Cook them without moving them for 2 to 3 minutes until the bottoms are browned. Then stir the tomato sauce in and add the capers, salt, olives, and artichoke hearts. Keep stirring and cooking this mixture for 2 to 3 more minutes, until shrimp are thoroughly cooked, and the artichoke hearts are hot.

3. To the sauce, add the drained cooked noodles and mix together.

4. To serve, divide the noodles and sauce between 4 plates or bowls. Enjoy!
5.

Low-Carbohydrate Variation: Use cooked spaghetti squash or cooked zucchini ribbons instead of linguini.

Low-Sodium Variation: Eliminate the table salt and kalamata olives.

Appetizer/Snack Selections

Flatbread Pizza with Spinach and White Bean Pesto

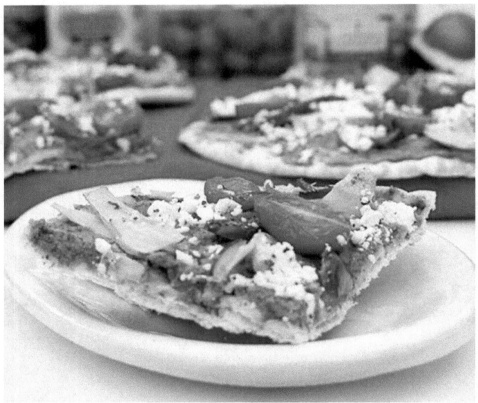

Total Prep and Cooking Time: 20 minutes

<u>Nutrition (per ½ flatbread for an appetizer; double for whole flatbread as a meal)</u>
Calories: 225
Fat: 9.5 g.
Carbohydrates: 28.5 g.
Protein: 8.5 g.

Serves 6 people for an appetizer or 3 people for a meal

If you have an intense desire for a pizza, rejoice! There's a nutritious, relatively guilt-free option that fits well in your Mediterranean eating plan. These delicious little flatbread pizzas should satisfy your craving without adding to your waistline. They're great as a main dish for a Friday night meal or served as an appetizer at a party. This dish piles on the produce, and the white bean and spinach pesto give this dish a unique flavor that will have your guests clamoring for more.

Components:
3 pieces of naan or pita bread (about 78 g. each, preferably whole-wheat)

2/3 c. canned cannellini or great northern beans, rinsed and drained

2 cups of spinach

1 Tbsp. Extra-Virgin olive oil

¼ cup raw natural almonds

¼ c. fresh basil, torn into pieces

2 T. water

¼ teaspoon salt, and additional for sprinkling

1/8 teaspoon black pepper

½ c. of cherry or grape tomatoes halved

½ c. marinated artichoke hearts, roughly chopped

½ of a medium avocado, sliced thinly

¼ small red onion, sliced thinly

2 oz. feta cheese with Mediterranean herbs

Preparation:
1. Turn on oven and set to 350 degrees Fahrenheit. On a baking sheet, place the 3 pieces of pita bread or naan.
2. In a food processor, add the following components: salt, pepper, water, basil, white beans, spinach, almonds, and basil. Pulse to puree until almost entirely smooth. Using a spoon, spread this pesto evenly on the pieces of bread.

3. Arrange the following on top of the pesto: onion slices, avocado slices, chopped artichoke hearts, and halved tomatoes. Sprinkle the cheese and a little salt over the top of each.
4. Place pan in the oven and leave it to bake for approximately 10 minutes, or until bread is crispy. Let it cool off slightly, then slice each flatbread into 4 pieces with a pizza cutter. Serve and enjoy!

Low-Carbohydrate Variation: Serve toppings on a low-carb crust or make a crust from pureed cauliflower.

Low-Sodium Variation: Eliminate the table salt. Substitute mozzarella for feta cheese. Use canned or frozen artichoke hearts instead of marinated.

Turkey Meatballs with Yogurt Herb Dip

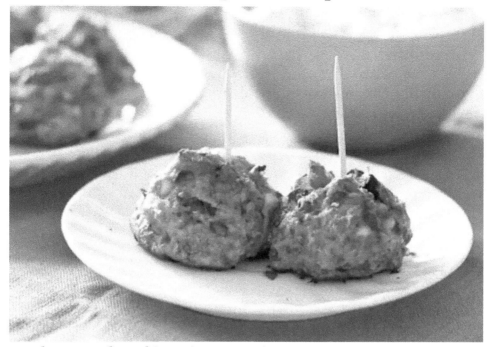

Total Prep and Cooking Time: 50 minutes

<u>Nutrition (per 2 meatballs)</u>
Calories: 157
Fat: 6.6 g.
Carbohydrates: 11.9 g.
Protein: 12.7 g.

The recipe makes 20 (2" diameter) meatballs.

These delightful little meatballs have a surprising twist – they have lentils, feta, and a few other unusual ingredients inside, the result of which is a perfect savory appetizer. In case you're wondering, they'd also be perfect in a batch of marinara sauce on pasta or mixed up with greens for a protein-packed salad.

Although they're hardly traditional, they contain several critical elements of the Mediterranean diet.

Components
For the meatballs
1 c. lentils, already cooked (black or green)
½ lb. ground turkey
2 lg. eggs, beaten
2/3 cup breadcrumbs
½ c. part-skim ricotta
¼ c. feta cheese crumbles
2 Tbsp. red onion, minced
2 Tbsp. black olives, chopped
1 Tbsp. capers
2 Tbsp. Italian parsley, minced
½ teaspoon oregano
¼ teaspoon dried dill
½ teaspoon of salt

For the yogurt dip
1 c. Greek yogurt (plain, nonfat)
1 clove of garlic, minced
½ teaspoon chives, fresh or dried
1 tsp. chopped dill, fresh or dried
1 teaspoon lemon juice
salt and pepper, as much as desired

Preparation:
1. Use a food processor to pulse cooked lentils until they have the consistency of mush, then move them from the food processor and place within a bowl. Then add the rest of the meatball components to the mushed-up lentils. Use your hands, a spatula, or a spoon to mix it all together thoroughly. Allow this mixture to rest for 15 minutes.

2. Heat up the oven and set it to 375 degrees Fahrenheit. Prepare a baking sheet with parchment paper or non-stick spray. Form 20 meatballs by hand from the meatball mixture and place them on the prepared baking sheet. They can be fairly close together because they don't spread out much.

3. Place the sheet of meatballs on the middle rack of the heated oven and bake them 20-22 minutes. They should be golden brown before you take them out of the oven. Allow them to cool off outside the oven.

4. While the meatballs bake, make the yogurt dip. Add all the components of the sauce to a small bowl and whisk them together until thoroughly combined. Cover the bowl and chill until ready to serve.

5. Keep meatballs and yogurt in the refrigerator until ready to serve. The meatballs will keep for 3 to 4 days, and the dip will keep for 7 to 10 days.

6. Enjoy!

Low-Carbohydrate Variation: This is a low-carb recipe. You can use more lentils and fewer breadcrumbs if you like, but this may change the texture too much.

Low-Sodium Variation: Eliminate the table salt. Use mozzarella instead of feta cheese.

Garlicy Spanish Shrimp

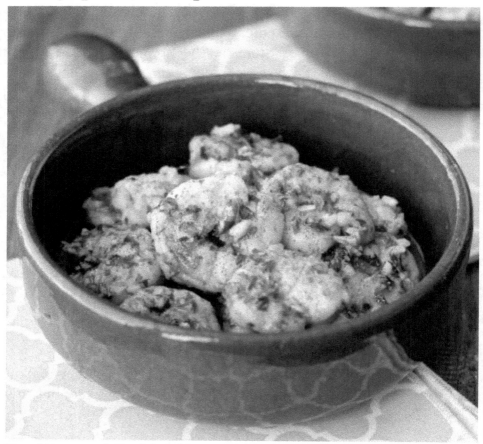

Total Prep and Cooking Time: 15 minutes

<u>Nutrition (per ¼ recipe)</u>
Calories: 250
Fat: 17.9 g.
Carbohydrates: 3.4 g.
Protein: 15.8 g.

Recipe serves 4 or more people.

Hardly anything beats shrimp when it comes to versatility and flavor delivered in a small package. This dish mimics the idea of Spanish *tapas* – small dishes designed to be shared between a few people. If you add toothpicks to the shrimp, you have a perfect snack or before-dinner appetizer. A bonus is all the nutrition packed into this dish. Shrimp deliver a large dose of selenium, which is an important nutrient for your immune system and heart. The olive oil adds some heart-healthy monounsaturated fat as well.

Components:
1/3 cup extra-virgin olive oil
4 cloves of garlic, minced
¼ teaspoon chili flakes
1 lb. large shrimp, deveined and peeled
1 teaspoon paprika
¼ teaspoon salt
1/8 teaspoon black pepper
2 Tbsp. dry sherry
1 ½ Tbsp. lemon juice
2 Tbsp. fresh parsley, chopped

Preparation:
1. To a large sautéing pan, add the oil, garlic and chili flakes. Set the heat under the pan to medium-high. Heating the oil with the garlic and chili will infuse the oil with these flavors. Be sure not to let the garlic brown.
2. After the oil becomes hot, place the shrimp in the pan and sprinkle the paprika, salt, and pepper over them. Stir the pan often while the shrimp cook for two minutes, until starting to turn pink.
3. Add the sherry and lemon juice to the pan. Keep stirring and cooking for another 2-3 minutes or until the shrimp are cooked through, and the liquid has reduced.

4. Sprinkle the parsley on top of the shrimp and serve. Enjoy!

Low-Carbohydrate Variation: This is a low-carbohydrate recipe.

Low-Sodium Variation: Eliminate the table salt.

Italian-Style Roasted Veggies and Mushrooms

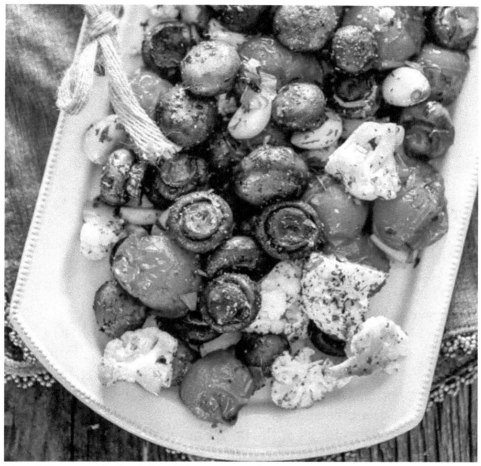

Total Prep and Cooking Time: 30 minutes

Nutrition (in each serving)
Calories: 87
Fat: 4 grams
Carbohydrates: 9 grams
Protein: 3 grams

Serves 6 people.

This simple dish makes a great appetizer or side dish. It's full of colorful, nutritious vegetables and sure to be a hit. Because it is so quick and easy to prepare, you'll love bringing it along to your next potluck party. Your waistline will appreciate the low-calorie count, too!

Components:
1 lb. cremini mushrooms, cleaned
2 c. cauliflower, cut into small florets
2 c. cocktail tomatoes
12 cloves garlic, peeled
2 Tbsp. extra-virgin olive oil
1 Tbsp. Italian seasoning
salt and pepper, as much as desired
1 T. fresh parsley, chopped

Preparation:
1. Turn on oven and set it to 400 degrees Fahrenheit.
2. Place all the mushrooms and vegetables within a bowl. Then include the olive oil, Italian seasoning, salt, and pepper. Use a spoon to toss until all these components are combined gently.
3. Spread contents of the bowl out on a sheet for baking and place it in the hot oven. Allow vegetables and mushrooms to roast 20 or 30 minutes. Make sure that the mushrooms are golden-brown (but not burnt) and the cauliflower can be easily pierced by a fork.
4. Sprinkle chopped fresh parsley over the dish just before serving. Enjoy!

Low-Carbohydrate Variation: The only carbohydrates in this dish come from vegetables, which cannot be eliminated without changing the recipe entirely.

Low-Sodium Variation: Eliminate the table salt.

Antipasto Skewers

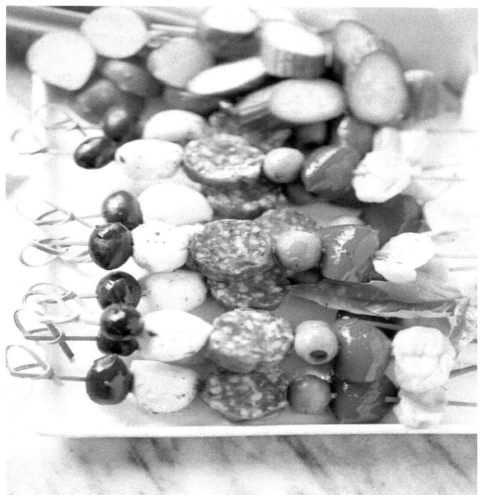

Total Prep and Cooking Time: 6 minutes

Nutrition (per skewer)
Calories: 55
Fat: 4 g.
Carbohydrates: 1 g.
Protein: 2 g.

The recipe makes 12 skewers.

These delicious and adorable little skewers take mere minutes to assemble, and they are sure to be a hit at your next party! They contain all the essential flavors of a Mediterranean diet, plus their small size makes portion control a cinch. The strong taste and unique texture of each bite are sure to satisfy you and your guests.

Components:
12 of each of the following
- kalamata olives, pitted
- mozzarella cheese balls
- small thick slices of salami
- pimento-stuffed green olives
- halves of jarred cherry peppers (6 peppers, cut in half)
- small pepperoncini peppers

Preparation:
1. Use 12 7-inch skewers. Stick one of each component on each skewer in any order of your choosing.
2. Store skewers in the refrigerator until ready to serve. These can be stored for up to a day.
3. Serve and enjoy!

Low-Carbohydrate Variation: This is a low-carb recipe.

Low-Sodium Variation: Unfortunately, most of the components of this recipe have a high level of sodium, so it is best to avoid this appetizer.

Conclusion

Thank for making it through to the end of *"Mediterranean Diet for Beginners."* Let's hope it was informative and able to provide you with all of the tools you need to achieve your healthy lifestyle goals.

By reading this book, you have made an essential first step in the exciting journey towards better health and a celebration of living with a fresh new approach to food. Now, you have the secret to why so many people around the Mediterranean Sea are living long, healthy, and happy lives surrounded by family members and friends. So, what are you going to do now that you know the secret?

The next step is to get cooking! Start shopping and cooking as soon as possible. You are likely eager to try some of the delicious recipes you read in this guide. If you are looking for more support, there are thousands of people online and throughout your community who have also embraced the Mediterranean lifestyle, and they will be eager to support you as you explore this new way of eating and approaching life. You'll also want to lace up your walking shoes and start getting active today. The sooner you start, the closer you'll be to achieving your goals of establishing and maintaining a healthy new lifestyle. You are at an exciting new place in life, so enjoy every moment of it!

Finally, if you found this book useful in any way, a review on Amazon is always appreciated!

CPSIA information can be obtained
at www.ICGtesting.com
Printed in the USA
LVHW020955301020
670159LV00012B/379